Primary Angle Closure Glaucoma (PACG)

Clement C. Y. Tham

Editor

Primary Angle Closure Glaucoma (PACG)

A Logical Approach in Management

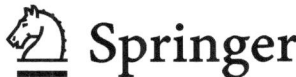 Springer

Editor
Clement C. Y. Tham
Department of Ophthalmology and Visual Sciences
The Chinese University of Hong Kong, Hong Kong Eye Hospital
Hong Kong SAR
China

ISBN 978-981-15-8122-9   ISBN 978-981-15-8120-5   (eBook)
https://doi.org/10.1007/978-981-15-8120-5

This Springer imprint is published by the registered company Springer Nature Singapore Pte Ltd. The registered company address is: 152 Beach Road, #21-01/04 Gateway East, Singapore 189721, Singapore

Foreword

Angle closure is a cause of more preventable blindness in the world than is open-angle glaucoma. I say that not as a pronouncement of faith but just because that is how the statistics have been presented over the past decade. Before I comment on this excellent and needed text, however, allow me to put in some background on the subject, because over the past years, it has been underdiagnosed or unrecognized and a subject of significant controversy in academic circles.

Earlier controversies, beginning in the nineteenth century, involved the mechanisms of aqueous production and outflow. Prior to the twentieth century, angle-closure glaucoma as a distinct entity was unknown. Well into the twentieth century, glaucoma was divided into two broad categories based upon its clinical presentation. Congestive, or inflammatory, glaucoma was characterized by conjunctival hyperemia and corneal edema, often accompanied by pain, and was divided into acute and chronic forms. Noncongestive glaucoma was characterized by a quiet eye and included both chronic open-angle glaucoma and chronic angle-closure glaucoma.

In 1856, von Graefe performed the first successful large surgical sector iridectomy for congestive glaucoma. This became the standard treatment for acute congestive glaucoma, although it was not always successful. It has little resemblance to the modern iridectomy, as glaucoma was thought to be caused by oversecretion of aqueous humor by the iris, and a large portion of the iris, thought responsible for aqueous production, was torn from its root. Over the second half of the nineteenth century, it was gradually realized that the ciliary body was responsible for aqueous production, that chronic inflammation pushed the iris forward and led to PAS, and that the effect of iridectomy was to open a closed angle.

At the turn of the twentieth century, several ophthalmologists suggested that iridectomy allowed increased communication between the posterior and anterior chamber. Nevertheless, because of a poor understanding of the pathophysiology, iridotomy and iridectomy were largely abandoned in favor of filtration procedures. Alexios Trantas developed gonioscopy and produced voluminous, highly accurate drawings of anterior segment conditions, but was largely ignored. It was not until the discovery of pupillary block and the development of peripheral iridectomy as a definitive procedure that a rational approach to the treatment of angle-closure glaucoma began. Edward Curran, at the University of Kansas, was the first to prove that obstruction of aqueous flow from the posterior to the anterior chamber led to the development of acute angle closure, and described relative pupillary block, its recognition, and treatment with peripheral iridectomy. He was not just ignored, but attacked and ridiculed. In 1931, he presented 500 cases and divided angle closure into acute and chronic with deep or shallow anterior chambers. Iridotomy was successful in acute attacks with iris bombe. The hostile reception continued.

It was not until 1948 that the AAOO divided glaucoma into wide or narrow angles with "vasomotor disturbances" in the ciliary body leading to angle closure. In 1952, Chandler accepted the concept of pupillary block and published extensively on its course and treatment, fully acknowledging Curran. Others in the USA accepted this, but it was not until the 1960s and development of the Goldmann lens freed gonioscopy from specialized clinics that Goldmann finally convinced François. However, Duke-Elder died never believing in gonioscopy, pupillary block, or iridectomy. In the 1960s, Ronald Lowe in Australia described ocular biometry and elucidated further the mechanisms of angle closure, while Mapstone in England devised provocative testing. In the 1970s, the development of laser iridotomy and, in the 1980s, laser iridoplasty for persistent angle closure after iridotomy and treatment of acute angle closure led to the beginning of the current era of greatly renewed interest in angle closure, its recognition, prevention, and successful management.

Current improvement in knowledge of genetic factors involved in various anterior segment anatomic parameters, including lens vault, iris thickness, plateau iris, and angle configurations, has improved knowledge of causation of angle closure. Great inroads have been made, particularly in East Asia, where angle closure remains characteristically most common, in the ability to diagnose and treat it. The lack of sufficient adeptness at gonioscopy and adequate laser facilities, especially in rural areas, led to the adoption of lens extraction (both clear and cataractous) to open the angle. This approach is now spreading to Europe and the Americas, although controversy remains as to when and under what conditions it should be performed for the greatest patient benefit.

Thus, this book is a timely essentiality to consolidate understanding of recognition of angle closure, understanding of mechanisms, and a variety of current and development modalities of management. Written by leading experts in the field, and not unexpectedly primarily from East Asia, the chapters span topics from a logical approach to management and objective quantitative evaluation of angle closure, to medical, laser, and surgical treatment, including lens extraction and goniosynechialysis (a modality I think much underused in the West), to filtering surgery, cyclodestruction, and MIGS, continuing on finally to other newer surgical options, management of acute primary angle closure, and continuing understanding of the underlying genetics and where and where not genetic factors may be applicable. It is a work in development, as progress continues apace in these areas, and this book provides a thorough and comprehensive work from which all ophthalmologists would benefit.

Robert Ritch
Einhorn Clinical Research Center, The New York Eye
and Ear Infirmary of Mount Sinai
New York, NY, USA

Scientific Advisory Board, The Glaucoma Foundation
New York, NY, USA

Preface

The conception of this textbook has arisen from an instruction course that has been jointly presented by a group of very dedicated glaucoma subspecialists, with expertise and experience in diagnosing, treating, and studying angle-closure diseases, since 2009. In its earliest days, this instruction course was presented under the auspices of the South East Asia Glaucoma Interest Group (SEAGIG). When the Asia-Pacific Glaucoma Society (APGS) was founded at the APAO Congress in Sydney in March 2011, SEAGIG was incorporated into APGS. Since then, this instruction course has become one of the important international educational programs of APGS. Over the years, this instruction course has been presented in innumerable international clinical ophthalmology conferences, including the Asia-Pacific Glaucoma Congresses (APGCs), the World Glaucoma Congresses (WGCs), the Asia-Pacific Academy of Ophthalmology Congresses (APAO Congresses), the World Ophthalmology Congresses (WOCs), and the Annual Meetings of the American Academy of Ophthalmology (AAO).

Through our interactions with clinical ophthalmologists from around the globe through these instruction courses, we appreciated the immense hunger for practical knowledge and skills in diagnosing angle closure, tips and pearls in laser and surgical treatments, as well as updates on the latest clinical, epidemiological, and basic science research on angle closure. We have also become aware that angle closure is frequently underdiagnosed, misunderstood, and occasionally mistreated, in some parts of the world. The authors do very much feel the pressing need to bring angle-closure diseases to the attention of the vast ophthalmological fraternity around the world.

Let me take this opportunity to thank all the authors who have contributed to this comprehensive and up-to-date textbook on primary angle-closure glaucoma and its management. Most of them have been participating regularly in the above APGS instruction course in the past decade, and in addition to being experts in angle closure, they are all key opinion leaders in this field as well as great teachers. I am very grateful to each of them for their selfless and immense contributions.

Last but certainly not least, I would express my deepest heartfelt thanks to Dr. Noel Chan, who has all along invested her time and energy to coordinate the preparatory work for this textbook. Without Noel's efforts, this textbook would not have been possible. Thank you, Noel!

Our understanding of angle closure and our management approach for this spectrum of diseases are ever evolving and advancing rapidly. We hope this textbook will allow readers to acquire a basic understanding of angle closure, and make good use of the practical knowledge and skills from this textbook in their daily clinical practice, for the greater benefit of their deserving patients.

Hong Kong, China   Clement C. Y. Tham

Contents

Primary Angle Closure Glaucoma (PACG): A Logical Approach Base on Angle Closures Types and Mechanism

Poemen P. Chan and Clement C. Y. Tham

Abstract

Primary angle closure disease is often regarded as one single disease entity in clinical management and research. However, angle closure is in reality due to different combinations of mechanisms in individual eyes, and these mechanisms include relative pupil block, plateau iris configuration, lens-related mechanisms, and also possibly increased choroidal pressure. These mechanisms often simultaneously contribute to the angle closure in a single eye, but with each mechanism contributing to varying extents in different eyes. In clinical practice and research, we often adopt one single intervention to reverse angle closure, without taking into consideration the predominant underlying mechanism leading to angle closure in each individual eye. Ideally, we should determine the most important mechanism predisposing each eye to angle closure, and then select the initial intervention (or combination of interventions) that can most effectively reverse this predominant mechanism with the least amount of surgical risks. Logically, the management approach should be individualized for each eye with primary angle closure disease, and the sequence of interventions should be logically based on the angle closure mechanism and type.

Keywords

Primary Angle Closure Glaucoma (PACG) · Relative pupil block · Plateau iris configuration · Lens related mechanism · Lens extraction · Laser Peripheral Iridotomy (LPI) · Argon Laser Peripheral Trabeculoplasty (ALPI)

P. P. Chan (✉)
Department of Ophthalmology and Visual Sciences, The Chinese University of Hong Kong, Hong Kong, SAR, China

Hong Kong Eye Hospital, Kowloon, Hong Kong, SAR, China
e-mail: poemenchan@cuhk.edu.hk

C. C. Y. Tham
Department of Ophthalmology and Visual Sciences, The Chinese University of Hong Kong, Hong Kong, SAR, China

Prince of Wales Hospital, Shatin, Hong Kong, SAR, China

Hong Kong Eye Hospital, Kowloon, Hong Kong, SAR, China
e-mail: clemtham@cuhk.edu.hk

Primary angle closure disease (PACD) may be further classified into primary angle closure glaucoma (PACG), primary angle closure (PAC), and primary angle closure suspect (PACS). The principle of treating PACD is to first reverse the anatomical angle closure as far as possible, with the aim of controlling the intraocular pressure (IOP), in order to prevent glaucomatous progression and blindness. Several mechanisms predisposing an eye to angle closure have been identified, including (1) relative pupil block, (2) plateau iris configuration (ciliary body anomalies), and (3) lens-related mechanism (including both the thickness and the anteroposterior position of the crystalline lens), with relative pupil block being the most common mechanism [1, 2]. These mechanisms often coexist in the same eye and they elicit the angle closure with variable degree of contribution. This concept is graphically represented in Fig. 1.1. Each column along the x-axis represents different eyes with varying anatomical predisposition to angle closure. The different coloured segments represent different mechanisms of angle closure, namely pupil block, plateau iris configuration, lens position, and lens thickness; each of these contributing to different extents in different eyes. The taller the segment, the more the contribution of that mechanism in a particular eye. As these overall columns (the "risk columns") increase in height, the eye may eventually develop PACS, PAC, or PACG, with time. For instance, in "Eye 3", angle closure is mainly contributed by plateau iris configuration, which leads to PAC. In "Eye 4", PACG is mainly contributed by lens thickness, which leads to PACG. As the patient increases in age, lens thick-

ness and pupillary block increase in importance and contribution. Therefore, an eye that has initial anatomical predisposition to angle closure may eventually progress to develop PACS, PAC, or even PACG, with time and age.

A logical treatment approach is to select a procedure (or a combination of procedures) that could remove the greatest amount of anatomical predisposition (hence, the greatest height from the risk column), with the least surgical risk. Table 1.1 summarizes the laser and surgical interventions (including laser peripheral iridotomy (LPI), argon laser peripheral iridoplasty (ALPI), and lens extraction) that are targeted towards individual anatomical mechanism for angle closure. LPI effectively and safely eliminates pupillary block, the most common angle closure mechanism, but does not have significant effect on reversing plateau iris configuration or lens mechanisms. ALPI effectively reverses plateau iris configuration and the appositional angle closure secondary to plateau iris, but it generally has no effect on pupil block or lens-related mechanisms. Lens extraction completely eliminates lens-related mechanisms. Lens extraction with intraocular lens (IOL) implantation creates a huge space between the anterior lens surface and the iris, and hence it also effectively eliminates the pupil block, and may be useful in

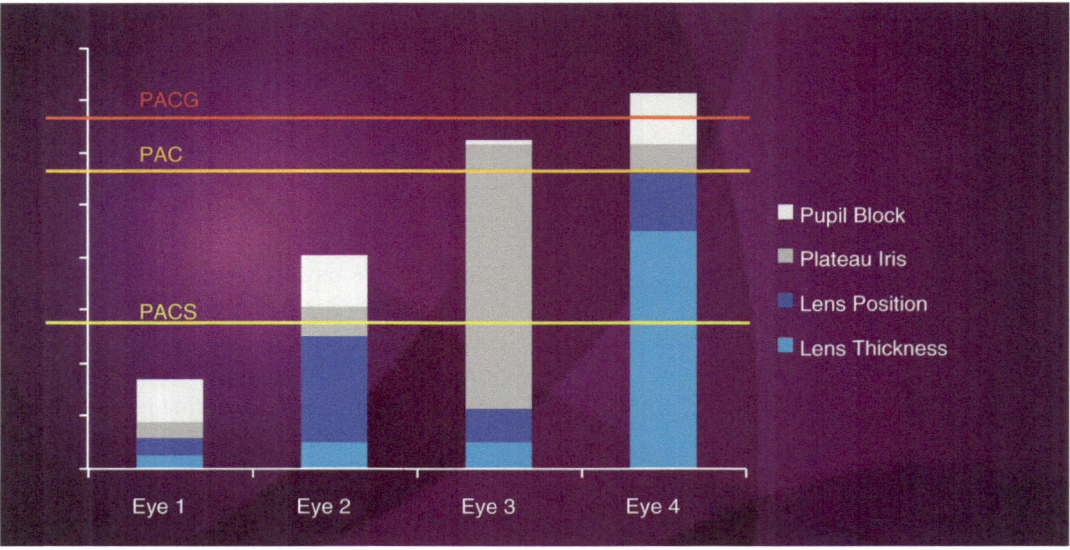

Fig. 1.1 Various combinations of angle closure mechanisms that lead to primary angle closure disease (PACD)

Table 1.1 Comparison of interventions that reverse anatomical predisposition to angle closure

Interventions reversing predisposition to angle closure	Interventions lowering IOP by bypassing blocked aqueous drainage	Intervention reducing aqueous production
• Laser peripheral iridotomy (LPI)[a] • Argon laser peripheral iridoplasty (ALPI)[a] • Lens extraction[a] • Goniosynechialysis (GSL)[b]	• Minimal invasive glaucoma surgery (MIGS) • Trabeculectomy and variations • Glaucoma drainage devices (GDD)	Cyclodestructive procedures • Cryotherapy • Diode laser transscleral cyclophotocoagulation (DLTSC) • Micropulse transscleral cyclophotocoagulation (MPTPC) • Endoscopic cyclophotocoagulation (ECP)

	Pupil block	Plateau iris	Lens position/thickness	Anterior synechiae	Relative risks	Visual benefit
LPI	+	−	−	−	++	−
ALPI	−	+	−	±	+	−
GSL	−	−	−	++	++	−
Lens extraction	+	±	+	+	+++	+

[a]Procedures that are specific for angle closure
[b]GSL could reverse anterior synechiae but could not eliminate the underlying angle closure mechanisms. Anterior synechiae is a consequence of angle closure rather than an initiating mechanism

reducing the contribution of plateau iris mechanism. The use of viscoelastic to expand the anterior chamber during phacoemulsification may also lead to a certain extent of peripheral anterior synechiae (PAS) breakdown (viscosynechialysis) and may contribute to further IOP reduction [3]. Lens extraction may, however, carry the highest surgical risk, as it is the only intraocular procedure amongst the three interventions. On the contrary, ALPI probably has the lowest risk because it requires lower laser power and energy compared to laser iridotomy.

Goniosynechialysis (GSL) involves the mechanical separation of the PAS. Unlike the 3 angle-opening procedures above, GLS alone does not reverse any of the underlying mechanisms of angle closure. Re-closure of the angle is possible after GSL, unless it is combined with another procedure that effectively reverses the anatomical predisposition to angle closure [4].

Visual improvement is another important consideration. Amongst the procedures above, lens extraction with IOL implantation is the only procedure that may offer visual improvement. Patients with good perceived visual acuity may be reluctant to undergo lens extraction surgery. Ophthalmologists may also be reluctant to remove an apparently clear lens. It should, however, be noted that a "clear" lens that contribute to angle closure should be considered pathological in nature, given its abnormal thickness or abnor-

mally anterior position in its anteroposterior axis, and it should be clearly explained to the patient that the lens removal could effectively remove the anatomical predisposition to angle closure in the eye. Clear lens extraction may also improve the patients' quality of life because of improved refractive outcomes, through IOL correction of significant hyperopia, astigmatism, and/or presbyopia. This is supported by the results of the EAGLE study, demonstrating that clear-lens extraction resulted in greater efficacy, better health status score, better visual quality, higher reduction of needs of medication, and prevent further glaucoma surgery when compared to LPI [5]. However, we should also keep in mind some of the limitations of the study [6, 7]. Prospective clinical trials have, in general, stringent inclusion criteria. A proven effective treatment may not be applicable to all patients with the same disease entity.

1.1 Treatment Algorithm for Angle Closure Disease

Figure 1.2a and b show two hypothetical situations of angle closure and explain how we may arrive at a logical treatment decision based on angle closure types and mechanisms.

Figure 1.2a is a hypothetical situation with 360° appositional angle closure with elevated IOP and glaucomatous optic neuropathy. In this scenario, if we assume that the trabecular meshwork and the drainage channels downstream from it have remained functional, we may only need to adopt an intervention (or a combination of interventions) to effectively reverse the anatomical predisposition to angle closure. Once the appositional angle closure is reopened, IOP control may be achieved, and further IOP-lowering interventions may not be necessary. If the patient has a visually significant cataract, cataract extraction would be the obvious first treatment choice, as it would both reopen the angle and improve vision. Supplementary ALPI could be considered if there is plateau iris configuration that leads to persistent appositional angle closure after the cataract extraction. If there is no visually significant cataract, LPI alone may be the choice of treatment if there is a significant pupil block. If there is persistent appositional angle closure with elevated IOP after LPI, one would need to identify the main underlying residual mechanism of angle closure and should select the appropriate next interventional step

accordingly (i.e. to perform ALPI if it is plateau iris syndrome, or to perform lens extraction if the angle closure is mainly due to lens mechanism). In the situation where both lens and plateau iris appear to be equally contributory, the decision would have to be made on a case-by-case basis, and with thorough discussion of the pros, cons, and risks of each option with the patient.

Figure 1.2b is another hypothetical situation with 360° complete synechial angle closure. The trabecular meshwork is sealed off by PAS. In this situation, the trabecular meshwork will remain sealed off if we conduct only measure(s) to reverse anatomical predisposition to angle closure. PAS is generally not disrupted by LPI or ALPI, even though it may be partly reversed by lens extraction, possibly through viscosynechialysis. To achieve IOP control, we may need additional surgical interventions that either disrupt the PAS (e.g. GSL), bypass the PAS (e.g. trabeculectomy), or reduce aqueous production (e.g. cyclophotocoagulation). Cataract extraction should be performed with or without additional IOP-

Fig. 1.2 (**a**) Treatment algorithm for eyes with a hypothetical 360° appositional angle closure with elevated intraocular pressure (IOP). (**b**) Treatment algorithm for eyes with a hypothetical 360° synechial angle closure with elevated intraocular pressure (IOP)

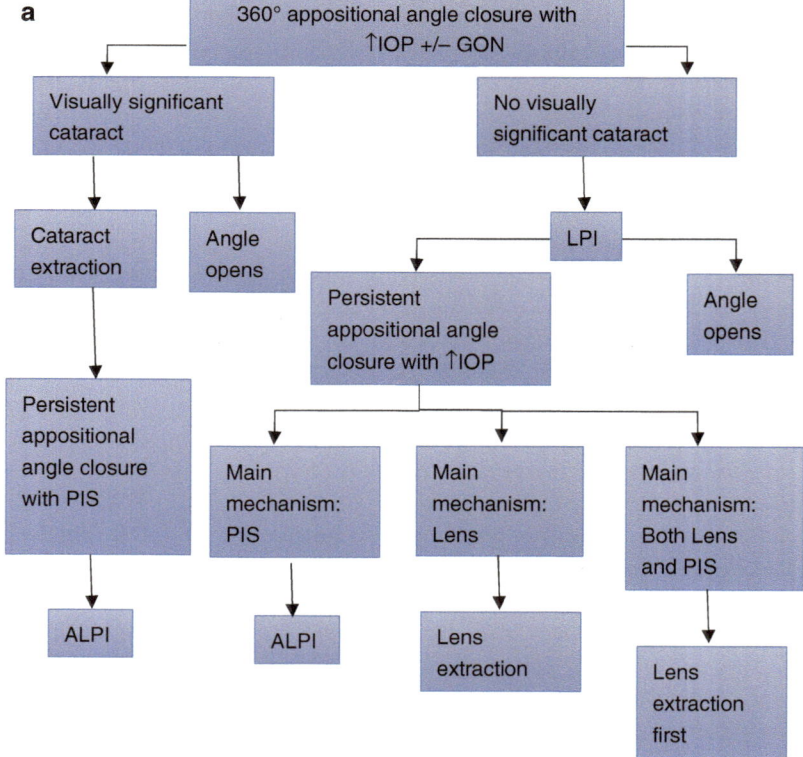

Fig. 1.2 (continued)

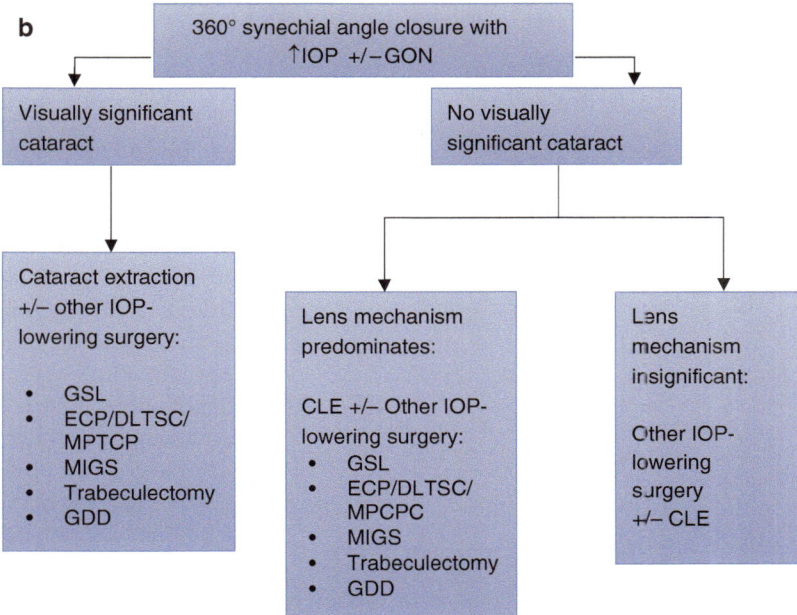

lowering procedures if the patients has visually significant cataract. Whether to perform additional IOP-lowering procedures depends on the IOP control and the severity of the glaucomatous optic neuropathy. If IOP is higher and a greater number of glaucoma drugs are in usage, in an eye with more severe and/or more rapidly progressive glaucomatous neuropathy, additional IOP-lowering procedures are more likely needed. The choice of procedure depends on the individual patient's circumstances and surgeon's expertise/ preference. If there is no visually significant cataract, we need to decide whether the lens mechanism is the predominating factor. If this is so, lens extraction may be considered, with or without other IOP-lowering procedures. If the lens is not the main mechanism, one may consider other IOP-lowering procedures first, with or without lens extraction.

1.2 Clinical Evidence of Plateau Iris Configuration and Lens Mechanism

Careful clinical examination and investigations are required to identify the underlying mechanism of angle closure. Gonioscopy, ultrasound

biomicroscopy (UBM), and to a certain extent, anterior segment optical coherence tomography (ASOCT), are important tools.

Plateau iris configuration describes the anatomical appearance in which the iris root angulates forward and centrally, which pushes the peripheral iris towards the trabecular meshwork, and thus narrowing or even closing the angle. Plateau iris syndrome (PIS) is defined as the development of angle closure in an eye with plateau iris configuration despite a patent iridotomy, with a subsequent increase in IOP. The diagnosis can be confirmed by darkroom gonioscopy, with the presence of the "double hump" sign on indentation gonioscopy, and UBM. ALPI is an effective procedure to revere plateau iris configuration. ALPI involves the application of large laser contraction burns at the peripheral iris, with a laser setting that is of long duration, low power, and of large spot size. This contracts the iris stroma at the site of the laser burns and allows the peripheral iris to be mechanically "pulled away" from the trabecular meshwork, which physically opens up the angle. Details of ALPI are described in Chap. 8. Endoscopic cyclophotocoagulation (ECP) reduces aqueous production, but at the same time shrinks ciliary processes and can thus at least partially reverse the angle closure caused

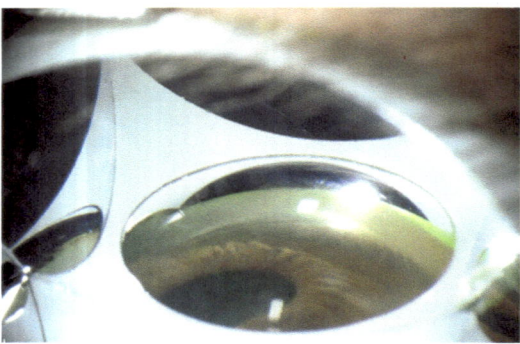

Fig. 1.3 The volcano-like appearance of the anterior surface of the iris–lens diaphragm, or "Mount Fujiyama" sign, in an angle closure eye in which the lens is the main mechanism leading to angle closure (gonioscopic view at slit lamp)

by plateau iris configuration [8]. Further study is required to confirm the effectiveness of ECP for the treatment of PIS.

For lens mechanism, the most important sign at the slit lamp would be a shallow central anterior chamber depth, which is the direct consequence of an abnormally thick crystalline lens and/or an anteriorly positioned lens. Unlike peripheral anterior chamber depth, the central anterior chamber depth is not influenced by the other mechanisms of angle closure (pupil block and plateau iris configuration). When performing gonioscopy at the slit lamp, the anterior surface of the iris–lens diaphragm may take on a volcano-like appearance, especially when the pupil is relatively constricted, and this is sometimes called the "Mount Fujiyama" sign (Fig. 1.3). This is a direct result of the iris draping over an anteriorly positioned and thick lens.

1.3   Summary

The authors aim to provide a management algorithm for treating PACD that is based on angle closure type and mechanism. Careful examination and investigation to identify the greatest contributing mechanism of angle closure would help ophthalmologist to select the treatment

intervention, or combination of interventions, that can most effectively reverse the anatomical predisposition to angle closure with the least amount of risk. This approach alone may often be sufficient in eyes with largely appositional angle closure. However, in eyes with largely synechial angle closure, additional IOL-lower procedures may be necessary to eliminate or bypass the PAS, or to reduce aqueous production, in order to achieve good IOP control.

Existing knowledge and investigational tools may not allow us to quantitatively evaluate the contribution of each individual mechanism, but we believe this framework should be useful for making logical clinical decisions for PACD patients, as well as in designing future interventional clinical trials for PACD.

References

1. Lowe RF. Anterior lens curvature. Comparisons between normal eyes and those with primary angle-closure glaucoma. Br J Ophthalmol. 1972;56:409–13.
2. Lowe RF, Clark BA. Radius of curvature of the anterior lens surface. Correlations in normal eyes and in eyes involved with primary angle-closure glaucoma. Br J Ophthalmol. 1973;57:471–4.
3. Lai JS, Tham CC, Chan JC. The clinical outcomes of cataract extraction by phacoemulsification in eyes with primary angle-closure glaucoma (PACG) and co-existing cataract: a prospective case series. J Glaucoma. 2006;15:47–52.
4. Lai JS, Tham CC, Lam DS. The efficacy and safety of combined phacoemulsification, intraocular lens implantation, and limited goniosynechialysis, followed by diode laser peripheral iridoplasty, in the treatment of cataract and chronic angle-closure glaucoma. J Glaucoma. 2001;10:309–15.
5. Azuara-Blanco A, Burr J, Ramsay C, et al. Effectiveness of early lens extraction for the treatment of primary angle-closure glaucoma (EAGLE): a randomised controlled trial. Lancet. 2016;388:1389–97.
6. Traverso CE. Clear-lens extraction as a treatment for primary angle closure. Lancet. 2016;388:1352–4.
7. Chan PP, Tham CC. Commentary on effectiveness of early lens extraction for the treatment of primary angle-closure glaucoma (EAGLE). Ann Eye Sci. 2017;2:21.
8. Hollander DA, Pennesi ME, Alvarado JA. Management of plateau iris syndrome with cataract extraction and endoscopic cyclophotocoagulation. Exp Eye Res. 2017;158:190–4.

Intraocular Pressure Fluctuation in Angle Closure Glaucoma

Prin Rojanapongpun, Anita Manassakorn, and Sunee Chansangpetch

Abstract

Angle closure glaucoma tends to have a higher magnitude and greater fluctuation of intraocular pressure (IOP), and thus leading to more blindness. Primary angle closure glaucoma (PACG) has higher IOP than other subtypes of angle closure and the normal subjects. The presence of PAS usually correlates with high IOP. The characteristic of diurnal IOP varies among the different subtypes of angle closure disease, greatest in PACG and smallest in primary angle closure suspect. However, the diurnal IOP fluctuation does not always characterize well in the different subtypes of angle closure disease. Cataract surgery, glaucoma laser procedure, and trabeculectomy in angle closure eyes potentially offer an advantage in flattening diurnal IOP curve. Some literatures suggest that greater 24-h diurnal IOP is associated with disease progression in this glaucoma entity, however, the available data are still limited and controversial. Nevertheless, diurnal IOP is worth exploring in PACG individuals who show glaucoma progression despite a favorable clinic visit IOP.

P. Rojanapongpun (✉) · A. Manassakorn
S. Chansangpetch
Glaucoma Research Unit, Department of Ophthalmology, Faculty of Medicine, Chulalongkorn University and King Chulalongkorn Memorial Hospital, Bangkok, Thailand

Keywords

Intraocular pressure fluctuation · Diurnal intraocular pressure · 24-h intraocular pressure · Angle closure glaucoma · Angle closure disease · Glaucoma progression

2.1 Intraocular Pressure and Angle Closure Glaucoma

Angle closure glaucoma (ACG) is less in number, but it blinds an equal number of people as open angle glaucoma (OAG) [1]. Compared with the rates of blindness in OAG, ACG has a threefold excess risk of severe bilateral visual impairment calculated from population-based studies [2]. The higher percentage of glaucoma blindness was also confirmed in hospital-based report [3]. As intraocular pressure (IOP) is a major risk factor for glaucoma progression, ACG likely has either a higher magnitude of IOP and its fluctuation.

There is enough evidence that ACG has higher diurnal IOP when compared to the normal non-ACG eye [4]. The range of IOP fluctuation was found to significantly increase with the severity or more advanced stage of ACG. The different clinical types of ACG can have different IOP profiles. Acute ACG usually has a very high IOP that abruptly rises during an acute attack. The IOP can remain high even after successful laser iridotomy (LPI). The main reason is that there may be other angle closure mechanisms, like plateau iris and lens mechanism, still operate in affecting the same eye [5, 6]. There is also a possibility that acute IOP rise damages the microstructures at the drainage angle as shown in a histopathological study [7]. This can be viewed as a structural damage of the trabecular meshwork after an acute attack and chronic structural damage in CACG in the area with or without pathological peripheral anterior synechiae (PAS).

The relationship between IOP and ACG is clear. The rise of IOP can be viewed as a functional loss of the anterior chamber drainage system and outflow facility. The formation of PAS and the histopathologic change of the trabecular meshwork can be viewed as a structural loss of the drainage angle. As ACG can blind more eyes than OAG, it is likely that the magnitude of IOP and its fluctuation is higher, especially if rapidly increased.

2.1.1   Angle Closure Subgroup and IOP

To better understand the relationship between ACG and IOP and its diurnal variation, one must have a clear picture of the different subgroups of ACG. Clinically, ACG can be classified into primary (PACG) and secondary ACG. However, based on the clinical presentation, it may be classified into acute, subacute, intermittent, and chronic ACG. Most of the recent publications classify ACG according to the International Society Geographical and Epidemiological Ophthalmology (ISGEO) into 3 subgroups: Primary angle-closure suspects (PACS), Primary angle-closure (PAC), and Primary angle-closure glaucoma (PACG). The PACS groups are those eyes in which the posterior trabecular meshwork was not visible for at least 180° on non-

indentation gonioscopy, with IOP of 21 mmHg or less and no optic nerve or visual field defect. The PAC eyes were those PACS who develops peripheral anterior synechiae (PAS) and/or raised IOP but without glaucomatous optic neuropathy. And PACG is PAC that develops structural and/or functional loss compatible with glaucoma. Such classification is essential as most of the studies did investigate the relationship of IOP to these different subgroups of ACG.

2.1.2   The Diurnal IOP in PACS, PAC, and PACG

Normal IOP variation ranged from 2 to 6 mmHg. The IOP is usually higher during the night-time because of the supine position and lower in the daytime due to the upright position [8]. Among the different subgroups of ACG who had LPI but without antihypertensive medications, a study using Goldmann applanation tonometer measured at 8 am, 12 pm, 4 pm, 8 pm, and 4 am found that PACG has the highest diurnal IOP of 7.38 ± 2.83 mmHg when compared to PAC at 5.52 ± 2.29 mmHg, and the PACS at 4.39 ± 1.47 mmHg [9]. Similar results were found in another study using noncontact air-puff tonometer measured every hour between 8 am and 5 pm, PACG showed high IOP fluctuation (5.4 ± 2.4 mmHg) compared to PAC (4.5 ± 2.3 mmHg), PACS (3.7 ± 1.2 mmHg) and normal controls (3.8 ± 1.1 mmHg). However, there was no significant difference between PACG and PAC groups. The highest IOP was found in the early morning. The extent of PAS and visual field loss pattern standard deviation (PSD) were associated with greater IOP fluctuation [10]. A significant difference between the peak diurnal IOP was also noted between the 3 subgroups with a strong correlation between peak IOP and its fluctuation. Peak IOP was higher out of the office hour in the majority of subjects with angle-closure [7]. Both studies were done by Asians, namely Indian and Chinese. These numbers may be less than the actual range of IOP fluctuation as it is not ethical to study the natural course of ACG without initial treatment of LPI or other therapy. In addition, both studies use instruments that need to measure in an upright position, therefore they may miss the IOP in a supine position or a habitual position. And not all time points were measured, i.e., no IOP data after 10 PM to before 7 AM. To be noted was that none of normal eyes had a diurnal IOP fluctuation of more than 6 mmHg together with any IOP reading more than 21 mmHg [4].

A higher diurnal IOP with a more advanced stage of ACG is conceivable by its classification. As the subgroups of PACG and PAC are defined by the high IOP or the development of PAS. As mentioned earlier, the high IOP can be viewed as functional damage of the aqueous drainage system at the anterior chamber angle. The formation of PAS can be viewed as structural damage of the drainage angle resulting from an adhesion between the peripheral iris and the trabecular meshwork. In other words, these are functional and structural losses in angle closure disease. The losses are extra to glaucomatous optic neuropathy but happening at the drainage angle where trabecular meshwork and outflow system resides. Clinically, the greater the amount of PAS, the higher the IOP fluctuation during office hours [11]. As PACS is a stage before any structural or functional change happens to the drainage angle, the diurnal IOP of PACS should be theoretically less than the more advanced stage of PAC and PACG, as well as not much different from the normal. This was shown in a study that the combined PACS and normal group had half the risk of IOP fluctuation of more than 3 mmHg when compared to the combined PAC and PACG group [8]. The office hours diurnal IOP fluctuation in asymptomatic PACS was less than that in treated PACG subjects and was

comparable to those treated PAC subjects. Moreover, greater IOP fluctuation was also associated with lens thickness and larger vertical cup to disc ratio [9]. It seems logical that eyes with PAS may have higher IOP than eyes without PAS. This is confirmed by another study using Goldmann applanation tonometer in PAC and PACS together with anterior segment optical coherence tomography (ASOCT) trying to find a relationship between smaller angle parameters and greater diurnal IOP fluctuation [12]. The study identified high IOP fluctuation to be correlated with many anterior segment OCT parameters, including AOD 750 (light), ARA 750 (light and dark), TISA 500 (light), TISA 750 (light), TIA 500 (light), and TIA 750 (light and dark). The IOP fluctuation could vary considerably from 1.5 to 14.5 mmHg. However, diurnal IOP fluctuation did not correlate well with PAS. But eyes with PAS are associated with higher IOP than eyes without PAS at each time point.

In acute primary angle closure, the IOP fluctuation was evaluated at least 3 months after LPI and compared with the fellow eye and the normal controls. The study used Goldmann applanation tonometer to measure every 2 hour between 9 AM to 11 PM. Eyes with a history of an acute attack had higher IOP at each time point, peak and trough, more than the normal group. However, there was no significant difference in terms of IOP fluctuation [13].

To summarize the characteristic of diurnal IOP in the different subtypes of angle closure disease. It is quite clear that PACG tends to have higher IOP than PAC, and PAC has higher IOP than PACS. The presence of PAS usually correlates with high IOP. However, the diurnal IOP fluctuation does not always characterize well in the different subtypes of angle closure disease. For a quick review, we summarize the results of IOP fluctuation, peak IOP, trough IOP, and mean IOP from various studies in Table 2.1.

Table 2.1 Summary of studies on IOP fluctuation, peak IOP, trough IOP, and mean IOP in different subtypes of angle closure disease

Authors (year)	IOP measurement period	Diagnosis	IOP fluctuation (mmHg)	Peak IOP (mmHg)	Trough IOP (mmHg)	Mean IOP (mmHg)
Gunning et al. (1998)	NA	PACG	11.5 ± 7.4	NA	NA	27.9 ± 8.1
Liu et al. (2006)	8 am–4 pm	PACS[a]	2.3 ± 1.7	NA	NA	14.4 ± 3.7
		PACG[a]	3.3 ± 2.5	NA	NA	14.3 ± 3.6
Baskaran et al. (2009)	8 am–5 pm	Normal	3.8 ± 1.1	15.9 ± 2.6	NA	13.9 ± 2.3
		PACS[a]	3.7 ± 1.2	16.0 ± 3.4	NA	13.9 ± 3.2
		PAC[a]	4.5 ± 2.3	20.0 ± 6.7	NA	17.6 ± 5.9
		PACG[a]	5.4 ± 2.4	20.1 ± 5.2	NA	17.0 ± 4.2
Sihota et al. (2010)	NA	PAC[a] with normal IOP	4.9 ± 1.5	20.1 ± 4.3	14.1 ± 3.3	20.8 ± 4.6
		PAC[a] with high IOP	6.3 ± 3.9	21.5 ± 4.5	15.1 ± 3.6	21.4 ± 4.4
		PACG[a]	5.8 ± 1.6	20.6 ± 1.1	15.2 ± 1.6	20.2 ± 3.0
Bhartiya et al. (2015)	8 am–4 am	PACS[a]	4.4 ± 1.5	18.2 ± 2.3	NA	15.9 ± 1.6
		PAC[a]	5.5 ± 2.3	21.9 ± 3.0	NA	18.8 ± 2.2
		PACG[a]	7.4 ± 2.8	25.7 ± 2.6	NA	21.3 ± 2.5
Park et al. (2015)	9 am–11 pm	Normal	2.7 ± 1.2	13.5 ± 2.3	10.9 ± 2.2	12.1 ± 2.2
		APAC[a]	2.5 ± 1.3	15.6 ± 4.2	13.1 ± 3.8	14.2 ± 4.0
		Fellow eye[a]	2.5 ± 0.8	14.4 ± 2.8	12.1 ± 2.7	13.1 ± 2.8
Sanchez-Parra et al. (2015)	9 am–4 pm	PAC/PACS	6.0 ± 2.7	20.0 ± 4.2	14.0 ± 2.8	18.5 ± 4.3
Ozyol et al. (2016)	8 am–4 pm	PACG[a]	4.2 ± 2.1	NA	NA	18.5 ± 4.2
Srinivasan et al. (2016)	8 am–5 pm	POAG	4.8 ± 1.7	17.2 ± 3.8	12.7 ± 3.1	16.5 ± 1.8
		PACS	3.6 ± 1.5	17.1 ± 2.3	13.5 ± 2.0	15.2 ± 2.5
		PAC[a]	4.5 ± 1.4	20.0 ± 3.0	15.5 ± 2.5	18.0 ± 2.0
		PACG[a]	4.6 ± 1.9	19.3 ± 3.1	14.7 ± 2.7	16.5 ± 1.8
Sihota et al. (2016)	7 am–10 pm	PAC/PACS	4.0 ± 2.1	NA	NA	14.4 ± 2.7

[a]With previous laser peripheral iridotomy

2.2 The Diurnal IOP of ACG Versus OAG

There is still conflicting evidence whether the diurnal IOP in ACG is greater than that of OAG. Factors responsible for the conflicts are whether the eyes were on treatment, how the diurnal IOP measurements were conducted, and the heterogeneous group of both entities. A study using Goldmann applanation tonometer measured every 3 hour from 7 am to 10 pm found higher IOP fluctuation in PACG (7.69 ± 3.03 mmHg) and POAG (8.31 ± 2.58 mmHg) as compared to normal (4.83 ± 2.46 mmHg). Nevertheless, there was no significant difference in magnitude between PACG and POAG. The ranges of IOP in both PACG and POAG were higher than the normal group (12–32 and 7–20 mmHg). The magnitude of IOP fluctuation of 6 mmHg or less was found in 15% of PACG and 9.3% of POAG, between 6 and 8 mmHg was found in 55% of PACG and

52% of POAG, and more than 8 mmHg was found in 30% of PACG and 38.6% of POAG. Therefore, IOP of more than 21 mmHg in combination with IOP fluctuation of more than 6 mmHg could be a good cutoff between normal and high fluctuation [4].

The time of peak IOP is still controversial. With Goldmann applanation tonometer, the peak IOP was found in the afternoon in PACG and normal groups, but POAG has peak IOP in the morning [4]. Another study using rebound tonometry to measure IOP every 4 hour from 8 am to 12 am in 1 week, the pattern of IOP fluctuation in PACG and POAG is similar. Both have peak IOP in the morning [14]. This is similar to another study using a noncontact air-puff tonometer [8].

It is still controversial in terms of trough IOP. Using rebound tonometry, the PACG group has a mean trough IOP greater than POAG [12]. However, the significant difference was not found in a study using Goldmann applanation tonometer (PACG; 17.8 ± 2.84 mmHg, POAG; 18.35 ± 2.51 mmHg) [4].

2.2.1 Effect of Cataract Surgery on 24-h IOP in ACG

There is plenty of evidence that cataract surgery can lower the IOP in POAG and PACG [15], and even in normal-tension glaucoma (NTG) [16]. One study showed that phacoemulsification could lower IOP by 13% and reduced glaucoma medications by 12% in POAG. However, for CACG, phacoemulsification reduced IOP by 30% and glaucoma medications by 58%. The hypotensive effect was even greater in patients with acute angle closure where a 71% reduction of IOP from the presentation and rarely required long-term glaucoma medications when phacoemulsification was performed soon after medical reduction of IOP. Even in PAC and PACG patients without cataracts, clear lens extraction could be more effective than LPI in reducing IOP and future glaucoma procedures [17]. However, the effect of cataract surgery on 24-h IOP is still controversial. A study in nonglaucoma subjects did not find the difference in the diurnal IOP fluctua-

tion after phacoemulsification and IOL implantation but only a significant reduction to mean IOP [18]. However, studies in NTG [19] and eyes with pseudoexfoliation [20] of both open and narrow angle eyes [21] demonstrated less IOP fluctuations after cataract surgery.

For angle closure eyes, removing lens means gaining more space in the anterior chamber and resulting in a less crowded anterior segment. The IOP lowering effect in these eyes could be substantial when compared to open angle eyes [22]. Cataract surgery is currently considered as one of the treatment options in angle closure disease [23]. But there are only a few studies exploring the relationship between diurnal IOP variation to cataract surgery in angle closure. As early as 1990, it was shown that extracapsular cataract extraction with intraocular lens (ECCE+IOL) could effectively lower IOP in both acute and chronic PACG [24]. It was later on reported that the IOP fluctuation in PACG eyes considerably reduced from 11.5 mmHg to 3.6 mmHg at approximately 1 year after ECCE+IOL [25]. The proportion of eyes that had the fluctuation of 8 mmHg or more was also reduced from 63.6 to 9.1%. It was shown that phacoemulsification with IOL significantly reduced daytime IOP fluctuation. Using Goldmann applanation tonometry to measure diurnal IOP during office hour at 3 months follow-up, the fluctuation reduced by 1.3 mmHg in PACG eyes but only 0.5 mmHg in PACS eyes [26]. A similar study found a significant reduction in IOP fluctuation from 4.58 mmHg to 2.84 mmHg at postoperative 2 months in PACG patients after phacoemulsification. Moreover, the analysis showed that the change in IOP fluctuation had a positive correlation with preoperative IOP fluctuation and postoperative increase in anterior chamber depth. And the change was independent of the preoperative mean IOP [27]. In contrast, another study using contact lens sensor to study 24-h IOP fluctuations and circadian IOP patterns of PACG patients before and 3 months after phacoemulsification, found no change in IOP fluctuation range but a significant decrease in the mean IOP and improvement of the anterior segment OCT angle parameters. Interestingly, only the range of the

IOP fluctuation during the nocturnal period was significantly decreased after the surgery [28]. One needs to be aware that the contact lens sensor does not measure the actual IOP but provides continuous monitoring of changes in the corneal curvature caused by IOP variation.

To summarize the effect of cataract surgery on IOP and its fluctuation. There is enough evidence that cataract surgery in PACG patient helps reducing IOP, and the need for hypotensive medication. There is suggestive evidence that cataract surgery may reduce the diurnal IOP, and preoperative IOP fluctuation could be a predictive factor.

2.2.2   24-h IOP in Post-trabeculectomy ACG

For POAG, there are evidence suggesting that trabeculectomy can lower peak IOP and IOP fluctuations in a greater amount than medical treatment [29, 30], especially in juvenile OAG patients [31]. This means that alternative aqueous drainage created in trabeculectomy can be a logical approach to a more uniform diurnal IOP.

As mentioned earlier, angle closure disease tends to have greater IOP fluctuation. Thus, trabeculectomy potentially offers an advantage in smoothening IOP curve, apart from lowering the mean IOP, in this group of patients. A study on an extended daytime IOP fluctuation (5 am–10 pm) of PACG patients after trabeculectomy showed a similar reduction to what has been described in POAG eyes receiving trabeculectomy. The peak IOP was usually in the early morning, and the trough IOP was at night. The daytime diurnal IOP fluctuation was 3.8 mmHg at 3 months postoperative period and positively associated with the higher peak and mean IOP [32]. Although the study did not have preoperative data and not included the control group, the IOP fluctuation was approximately the same as what had been reported in normal subjects [33]. Interestingly, lesser IOP variation was demonstrated in eyes with a greater bleb extent and the presence of microcysts. In other words, the favorable functioning bleb appearance seems to offer flatter diurnal IOP. The study did not find a significant

association between IOP fluctuation and the degree of PAS, cup-to-disc ratio, and glaucoma visual field severity. This suggested that postoperative IOP variation was not influenced by preoperative severity of the disease.

2.2.3   Effect of Glaucoma Laser Intervention on 24-h IOP in ACG

At present, it is not known whether laser treatment in angle closure would influence the IOP fluctuation. It is known that LPI can deepen the anterior chamber and widen the angle, both of which can be objectively measured by anterior segment imaging [34, 35]. The widening of the angle facilitates the aqueous drainage through the conventional outflow pathway and may dampen the IOP fluctuation. Given the association between smaller angle parameters and greater IOP fluctuation [36], it has been speculated that LPI can decrease the magnitude of the fluctuation. However, current evidence of IOP fluctuation in angle closure disease is mostly obtained from eyes that already underwent laser iridotomy. A study that compared the IOP fluctuation between acute PAC eyes after iridotomy, fellow eyes after iridotomy, and normal controls, did not find the difference of IOP fluctuation among the three groups [37]. The study suggested that LPI did not have a significant effect on the diurnal IOP pattern. Another study evaluated the IOP before and 1 month after laser iridotomy in PACS and PAC patients. Although the diurnal variation decreased from 4.0 mmHg to 3.5 mmHg after the procedure, the difference did not reach a statistically significant level [38].

Laser peripheral iridoplasty can also widen the anterior chamber angle [39]. In contrast to the LPI, it was found that iridoplasty significantly decreased IOP fluctuation by 1.56 mmHg at 12 weeks after treatment in PAC and PACS subjects with gonioscopically occludable angles following LPI. In addition, comparing iridoplasty-treated versus the untreated eyes who had previous LPI, the results demonstrated that the difference in the IOP fluctuation mostly contributed to the drop of the maximum diurnal IOP after the laser rather than the change of the minimum diurnal IOP.

2.2.4 24-h IOP and ACG Progression

The role of 24-h diurnal IOP as an independent risk factor of glaucoma progression is still controversial. It has been speculated that the IOP fluctuation causes the mechanical stress to the lamina cribrosa (LC) [40, 41]. The repeated wear and tear processes subsequently lead to structural modification and stiffening of the LC. This remodeling may also further compromise the LC from the decrease of nutrient delivery from capillary [42]. Several studies concluded that IOP fluctuation led to the progression of glaucoma, especially in OAG. However, most studies were not specific to 24-h diurnal IOP. The Advanced Glaucoma Intervention Study (AGIS) suggested that greater IOP fluctuation increased risk factor for visual field progression in glaucoma [43]. Both diurnal and long-term fluctuations may contribute to glaucoma progression in susceptible populations [44]. In contrast, the data from the Early Manifest Glaucoma Trial (EMGT) did not support IOP fluctuation as an independent factor for progression [45]. Moreover, long-term IOP fluctuation does not appear to be an important risk for ocular hypertension to progress to glaucoma [46]. Another hospital-based study also suggested that diurnal IOP may be less important than the mean and peak IOP in OAG [47]. Based on a meta-analysis, which evaluated the association of IOP fluctuation and OAG progression, there was no statistical significance in short-term IOP fluctuation with glaucoma progression (HR 0.98 95% CI 0.78–1.24). Whereas the long-term fluctuation was a significant risk factor for the progression (HR 1.43 95% CI 1.13–1.82) [48]. The visual field defined the progression in the study with or without glaucomatous structural parameters.

For angle closure disease, there was a study using contact lens sensors during normal daily activities to evaluate the 24-h IOP fluctuation profile between progressing and stable PACG eyes [49]. The progression was determined by visual field mean deviation, visual field index, and retinal nerve fiber layer thickness. Although no statistically significant difference was observed in the overall IOP signal, the authors found larger IOP fluctuation in the progressive eyes compared to the stable eyes at specific time points during the bedtime hours (6 PM to 1 AM) and the wake-up hours (3 AM to 11 AM). The authors hypothesized that the larger IOP fluctuation in the progressive group during bedtime and wake-up hours might be due to greater response to the postural change. Thus, implying the possible relationship between ocular perfusion pressure and IOP. Another study of daytime diurnal IOP (8 AM to 5 PM) showed a wider diurnal IOP fluctuation of 4–5 mmHg in the PACG and PAC eyes. The range was greater than in the PACS subjects and the normal controls. The degree of PAS and visual field loss were associated with IOP fluctuation in PAC and PACG eyes [50].

Although there are some suggestive pieces of evidence that greater 24-h diurnal IOP associate with a greater chance of disease progression in ACG, yet still lack strong evidence to conclude that it is an independent risk factor for ACG progression. The same conclusion applies to OAG progression. Nevertheless, there is little doubt that peak and mean IOP associate with disease progression.

2.2.5 Risk Factors of 24-h IOP Fluctuation

Currently, the information on the risk factor that causes 24-h IOP fluctuation (including nocturnal IOP) in ACG is inadequate. There was a study looking at the association of daytime diurnal IOP fluctuation with various variables, including the extent of PAS, central corneal thickness, cup-to-disc ratio, and visual field pattern standard deviation [48]. Among these variables, only the extent of PAS and PSD had a significant association with greater daytime diurnal IOP fluctuation. With the definition of IOP fluctuation as the standard deviation of office-hour IOP measurements, another study found that the number of clock hours of PAS, lens thickness, cup-to-disc ratio were predictive factors associated with IOP fluctuation [9]. The presence of PAS can reflect the compromised trabecular meshwork function and thus results in greater IOP variation. Also, the thick lens occupies more space in the anterior chamber, which can obliterate the angle and interfere with the aqueous drainage. Noteworthy, both studies solely evaluated the daytime IOP (8 am–5 pm), and most eyes had already received LPI. Moreover, several factors, such as blood pressure, heart rate, systemic medication use, and postural change potentially affect the IOP fluctuation and need further explorations.

Anterior segment OCT was used to identify which angle parameter measurements may predict the magnitude of IOP diurnal fluctuations in PAC or PACS patients [10]. Greater daytime diurnal fluctuation was statistically significantly associated with AOD 750 (light), ARA 750 (light and dark), TISA 500 (light), TISA 750 (light), TIA 500 (light), and TIA 750 (light and dark). The higher IOP levels during the day are related to the circumferential extent of PAS. The results for diurnal IOP fluctuation suggested that an eye with smaller angle dimensions would exhibit a greater range of IOP, defined by the difference between peak and trough during the day. It was suggested that OCT angle parameter measurements could be used to predict IOP diurnal fluctuations in at-risk patients.

For long-term IOP fluctuation, which is not 24-h diurnal IOP, baseline IOP correlated positively with the fluctuation [51]. Although the degree of PAS showed a significant association in the univariate model, the factor did not reach a statistically significant level after adjusting the baseline IOP in the multivariate model. According to the study, neither baseline cup-to-disc ratio nor mean deviation on automated perimetry had an association with the long-term IOP fluctuation.

While there are needs to find the specific risk factors and good biomarkers of the 24-h diurnal IOP in ACG, the structural damage at the angle that characterized by PAS, and the functional damage of the drainage that characterized by high IOP seem to offer themselves some good clues for high 24-h diurnal IOP. This could lead to structural and functional damage of the optic nerve head (ONH) characterized by ONH changes and visual field losses (see Fig. 2.1). There is a necessity to conduct a few more studies that measure 24-h diurnal IOP and investigates different risk factors in different subtypes of angle closure.

2.2.6 Clinical Use of 24-h Diurnal IOP in ACG

There is always a question of whether 24-h diurnal IOP has clinical importance in the management of ACG. In principle, more information may lead to a

Fig. 2.1 Structural and functional damages of angle closure and glaucomatous optic neuropathy

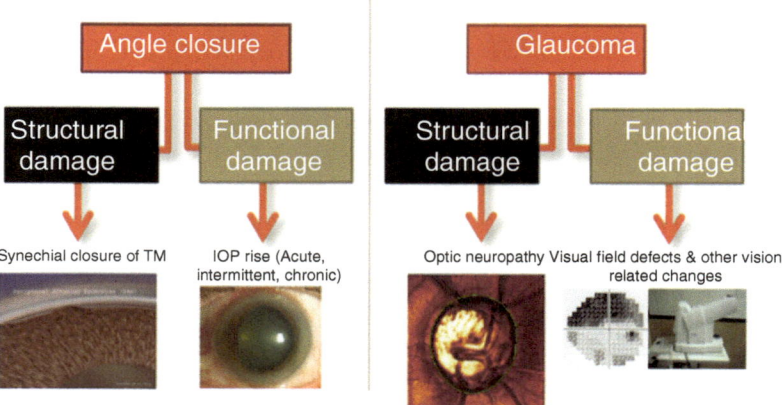

better decision. The potential clinical implication of 24-h IOP is that we have more information on the most important clinical risk factor of glaucomatous damage as there are more IOP data points than just a one-time IOP data point at each clinical visit. This could be a crucial assessment in PACG patients that progress despite a favorable clinic visit IOP. However, 24-h diurnal IOP recordings are a practical challenge for both the clinician and the patient. This could be very difficult for including nocturnal IOP recordings as more resources must be used. The usual practice requires hospital admission of patients overnight, and the effort of recording IOP during sleep can be strenuous in some patients. Furthermore, there is a controversy on whether IOP recordings should be taken before getting out of bed or after. Moreover, the rapid changes of IOP that occur over the first 10–15 min on waking could also be considerable. Therefore, most studies have investigated only daytime or office-hour IOP fluctuation.

Many studies skipped the nocturnal IOP measurements or the IOP measurements after midnight. So, this would lead to incomplete IOP profile and might miss IOP peaks at specific time points and for the habitual position. This could explain the variation in the timing of the IOP peak reported from the studies [2, 7–9, 47]. Based on the available evidence, 24-h diurnal IOP behavior cannot be adequately characterized by daytime or office-hour IOP assessment in ACG. For example, a retrospective study found that two-thirds of the primary adult-onset glaucoma patients had peak IOP measurements outside office-hour and diurnal IOP fluctuation was significantly higher than office IOP fluctuation [52]. We used rebound tonometry to study 24-h diurnal IOP in 40 PACG at their residents in habitual positions. We found that the peak IOP appeared at 3 am–6 am with the highest IOP fluctuation between 9 pm and midnight (unpublished data, Fig. 2.2). Even under medical treatment and LPI, more than half of PACG patients had high peak IOP and wide diurnal IOP outside office hours. We also studied a group of 41 age-matched POAG patients with the same number of glaucoma medications and visual field losses. The frequency of the peak IOP were also between

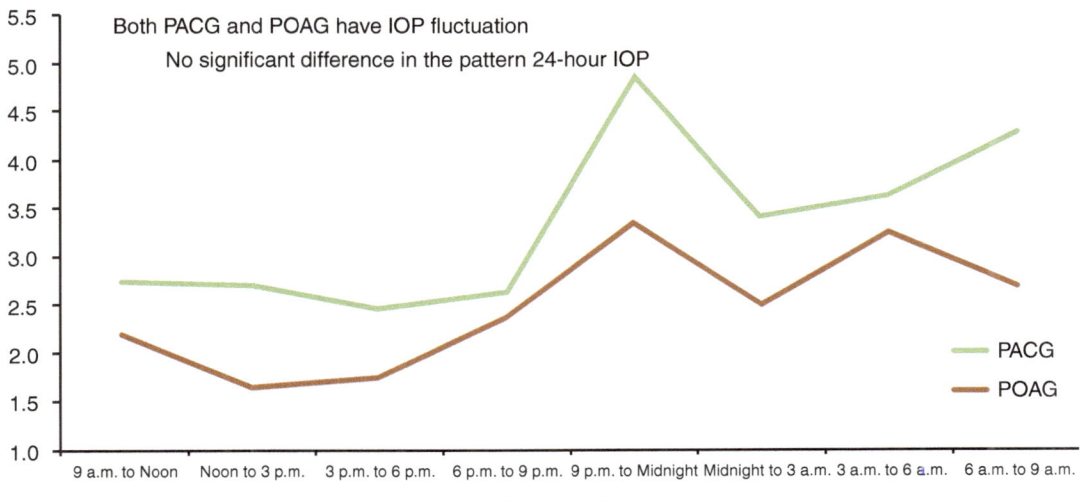

Fig. 2.2 Pattern of 24-h diurnal IOP in PACG and POAG

Fig. 2.3 The peak IOP
of the studied PACG and
POAG patients at the
different 24-h diurnal
IOP time point

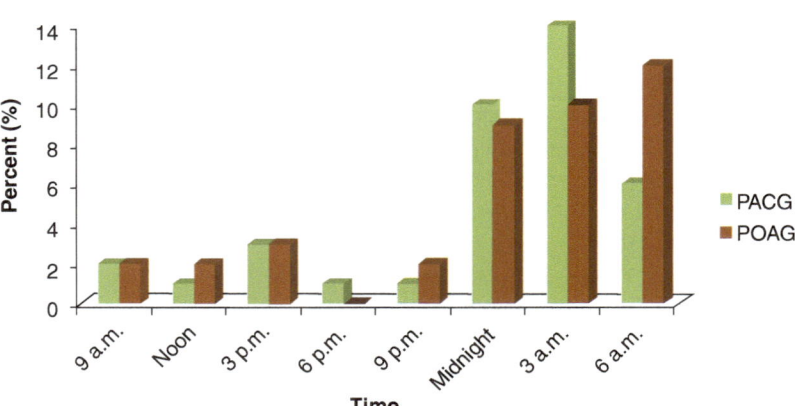

Distribution of peak IOP

midnight to 6 am with highest peak at 6 am but reduced thereafter (Fig. 2.3). The pattern of 24-h diurnal IOP was not significantly different between PACG and POAG. However, the peak IOP and the range of IOP fluctuation were slightly higher in PACG even under treatment.

In conclusion, office hours IOP poorly characterizes 24-h IOP because most PACG patients have peak IOP and higher fluctuation outside daytime IOP. In practice, selectively investigate into 24-h diurnal IOP, for individuals in whom seem to have good office IOP but progressing or of advanced damage with good IOP profiles, may provide a better guide to managing the patients properly. Until we have a reliable and an affordable 24-h diurnal IOP monitoring device or a specific biomarker of diurnal IOP, the practical approach is trying to measure IOP at the different time points in the clinic may help to identify those who may have a higher risk of IOP fluctuation and the necessity of further investigation and 24-h diurnal IOP.

References

1. Quigley HA, Broman AT. The number of people with glaucoma worldwide in 2010 and 2020. Br J Ophthalmol. 2006;90(3):262–7. https://doi.org/10.1136/bjo.2005.081224.
2. Friedman DS, Foster PJ, Aung T, He M. Angle closure and angle-closure glaucoma: what we are doing now and what we will be doing in the future. Clin Exp Ophthalmol. 2012;40(4):381–7. https://doi.org/10.1111/j.1442-9071.2012.02774.x.
3. Cronemberger S, Lourenço LF, Silva LC, Calixto N, Pires MC. Prognosis of glaucoma in relation to blindness at a university hospital. Arq Bras Oftalmol. 2009;72(2):199–204. https://doi.org/10.1590/s0004-27492009000200013.
4. Sihota R, et al. A comparison of the circadian rhythm of intraocular pressure in primary phronic angle closure glaucoma, primary open angle glaucoma and normal eyes. Indian J Ophthalmol. 2005;53:243–7. https://doi.org/10.4103/0301-4738.18905.
5. Nonaka A, et al. Cataract surgery for residual angle closure after peripheral laser iridotomy. Ophthalmology. 2005;112:974–9. https://doi.org/10.1016/j.ophtha.2004.12.042.
6. Lee KS, et al. Residual anterior chamber angle closure in narrow-angle eyes following laser peripheral iridotomy: anterior segment optical coherence tomography quantitative study. Jpn J Ophthalmol. 2011;55:213–9. https://doi.org/10.1007/s10384-011-0009-3.
7. Sihota R, et al. The trabecular meshwork in acute and chronic angle closure glaucoma. Indian J Ophthalmol. 2001;49:255–9.
8. Medical Advisory S. Diurnal tension curves for assessing the development or progression of glaucoma: an evidence-based analysis. Ont Health Technol Assess Ser. 2011;11:1–40.
9. Bhartiya S, Ichhpujani P. Diurnal intraocular pressure fluctuation in eyes with angle-closure. J Curr Glaucoma Pract. 2015;9:20–3. https://doi.org/10.5005/jp-journals-10008-1178.
10. Baskaran M, et al. Diurnal intraocular pressure fluctuation and associated risk factors in eyes with angle closure. Ophthalmology. 2009;116:2300–4. https://doi.org/10.1016/j.ophtha.2009.06.010.
11. Srinivasan S, et al. Diurnal intraocular pressure fluctuation and its risk factors in angle-closure and open-

angle glaucoma. Eye (Lond). 2016;30:362–8. https://doi.org/10.1038/eye.2015.231.

12. Sanchez-Parra L, Pardhan S, Buckley RJ, Parker M, Bourne RR. Diurnal intraocular pressure and the relationship with swept-source OCT-derived anterior chamber dimensions in angle closure: the IMPACT study. Invest Ophthalmol Vis Sci. 2015;56:2943–9. https://doi.org/10.1167/iovs.14-15385.

13. Park HS, et al. Diurnal intraocular pressure changes in eyes affected with acute primary angle closure and fellow eyes after laser peripheral iridotomy. Jpn J Ophthalmol. 2015;59:318–24. https://doi.org/10.1007/s10384-015-0399-8.

14. Tan S, et al. Comparison of self-measured diurnal intraocular pressure profiles using rebound tonometry between primary angle closure glaucoma and primary open angle glaucoma patients. PLoS One. 2017;12:e0173905. https://doi.org/10.1371/journal.pone.0173905.

15. Chen PP, et al. The effect of phacoemulsification on intraocular pressure in Glaucoma patients: a report by the American Academy of ophthalmology. Ophthalmology. 2015;122:1294–307. https://doi.org/10.1016/j.ophtha.2015.03.021.

16. Seol BR, et al. Intraocular pressure (IOP) change and frequency of IOP spike after cataract surgery in Normal-tension Glaucoma: a case-control Study. J Glaucoma. 2019;28:201–6. https://doi.org/10.1097/IJG.0000000000001172.

17. Azuara-blanco A, Burr J, Ramsay C, et al. Effectiveness of early lens extraction for the treatment of primary angle-closure glaucoma (EAGLE): a randomised controlled trial. Lancet. 2016;388:1389–97.

18. Kim KS, Kim JM, Park KH, Choi CY, Chang HR. The effect of cataract surgery on diurnal intraocular pressure fluctuation. J Glaucoma. 2009;18:399–402. https://doi.org/10.1097/IJG.0b013e3181879e89.

19. Tojo N, Otsuka M, Hayashi A. Comparison of intraocular pressure fluctuation before and after cataract surgeries in normal-tension glaucoma patients. Eur J Ophthalmol. 2019;29:516–23. https://doi.org/10.1177/1120672118801163.

20. Rao A. Diurnal curve after phacoemulsification in patients with pseudoexfoliation syndrome and cataract. Semin Ophthalmol. 2012;27:1–5. https://doi.org/10.3109/08820538.2011.626356.

21. Vahedian Z, et al. Pseudoexfoliation syndrome: effect of phacoemulsification on intraocular pressure and its diurnal variation. J Curr Ophthalmol. 2015;27:12–5. https://doi.org/10.1016/j.joco.2015.09.006.

22. Kim WJ, Kim JM, Kim KN, Kim CS. Effect of preoperative factor on intraocular pressure after phacoemulsification in primary open-angle Glaucoma and primary angle-closure Glaucoma. Kor J Ophthalmol: KJO. 2019;33(4):303–14. https://doi.org/10.3341/kjo.2018.0135.

23. Azuara-Blanco A, Burr J, Ramsay C, Cooper D, Foster PJ, Friedman DS, Scotland G, Javanbakht M, Cochrane C, Norrie J, EAGLE Study Group. Effectiveness of early lens extraction for the treatment of primary angle-closure glaucoma (EAGLE): a randomised controlled trial. Lancet (London, England). 2016;388(10052):1389–97. https://doi.org/10.1016/S0140-6736(16)30956-4.

24. Gunning FP, Greve EL. Uncontrolled primary angle closure glaucoma: results of early intercapsular cataract extraction and posterior chamber lens implantation. Int Ophthalmol. 1991;15(4):237–47. https://doi.org/10.1007/bf00171026.

25. Gunning FP, Greve EL. Lens extraction for uncontrolled angle-closure glaucoma: long-term follow-up. J Cataract Refract Surg. 1998;24(10):1347–56. https://doi.org/10.1016/s0886-3350(98)80227-7.

26. Liu CJ, Cheng CY, Wu CW, Lau LI, Chou JC, Hsu WM. Factors predicting intraocular pressure control after phacoemulsification in angle-closure glaucoma. Arch Ophthalmol (Chicago, Ill: 1960). 2006;124(10):1390–4. https://doi.org/10.1001/archopht.124.10.1390.

27. Özyol P, Özyol E, Sül S, Baldemir E, Çavdar S. Intraocular pressure fluctuation after cataract surgery in primary angle-closure glaucoma eyes medically controlled after laser iridotomy. Acta Ophthalmol. 2016;94(7):e528–33. https://doi.org/10.1111/aos.13023.

28. Tojo N, Otsuka M, Miyakoshi A, Fujita K, Hayashi A. Improvement of fluctuations of intraocular pressure after cataract surgery in primary angle closure glaucoma patients. Graefe's Arch Clin Exp Ophthalmol = Albrecht von Graefes Archiv fur klinische und experimentelle Ophthalmologie. 2014;252(9):1463–8. https://doi.org/10.1007/s00417-014-2666-7.

29. Medeiros FA, Pinheiro A, Moura FC, Leal BC, Susanna R Jr. Intraocular pressure fluctuations in medical versus surgically treated glaucomatous patients. J Ocul Pharmacol Ther: the official journal of the Association for Ocular Pharmacology and Therapeutics. 2002;18(6):489–98. https://doi.org/10.1089/108076802321021036.

30. Konstas AG, Topouzis F, Leliopoulou O, Pappas T, Georgiadis N, Jenkins JN, Stewart WC. 24-hour intraocular pressure control with maximum medical therapy compared with surgery in patients with advanced open-angle glaucoma. Ophthalmology. 2006;113(5):761–5.e1. https://doi.org/10.1016/j.ophtha.2006.01.029.

31. Park SC, Kee C. Large diurnal variation of intraocular pressure despite maximal medical treatment in juvenile open angle glaucoma. J Glaucoma. 2007;16(1):164–8. https://doi.org/10.1097/01.ijg.0000212278.03595.39.

32. Liang YB, Xie C, Meng HL, et al. Daytime fluctuation of intraocular pressure in patients with primary angle-closure glaucoma after trabeculectomy. J Glaucoma. 2013;22(5):349–54. https://doi.org/10.1097/IJG.0b013e31826a7dd5.

33. Baskaran M, Kumar RS, Govindasamy CV, et al. Diurnal intraocular pressure fluctuation and associated risk factors in eyes with angle closure.

Ophthalmology. 2009;116(12):2300–4. https://doi.org/10.1016/j.ophtha.2009.06.010.

34. Zebardast N, Kavitha S, Krishnamurthy P, Friedman DS, Nongpiur ME, Aung T, Quigley HA, Ramulu PY, Venkatesh R. Changes in anterior segment morphology and predictors of angle widening after laser Iridotomy in south Indian eyes. Ophthalmology. 2016;123(12):2519–26. https://doi.org/10.1016/j.ophtha.2016.08.020.

35. Zhekov I, Pardhan S, Bourne RR. Optical coherence tomography-measured changes over time in anterior chamber angle and diurnal intraocular pressure after laser iridotomy: IMPACT study. Clin Exp Ophthalmol. 2018;46(8):895–902. https://doi.org/10.1111/ceo.13303.

36. Sanchez-Parra L, Pardhan S, Buckley RJ, Parker M, Bourne RR. Diurnal intraocular pressure and the relationship with swept-source OCT-derived anterior chamber dimensions in angle closure: the IMPACT Study. Invest Ophthalmol Vis Sci. 2015;56(5):2943–9. https://doi.org/10.1167/iovs.14-15385.

37. Park HS, Kim JM, Shim SH, et al. Diurnal intraocular pressure changes in eyes affected with acute primary angle closure and fellow eyes after laser peripheral iridotomy. Jpn J Ophthalmol. 2015;59(5):318–24. https://doi.org/10.1007/s10384-015-0399-8.

38. Sihota R, Rishi K, Srinivasan G, Gupta V, Dada T, Singh K. Functional evaluation of an iridotomy in primary angle closure eyes. Graefe's Arch Clin Exp Ophthalmol = Albrecht von Graefes Archiv fur klinische und experimentelle Ophthalmologie. 2016;254(6):1141–9. https://doi.org/10.1007/s00417-016-3298-x.

39. Bourne R, Zhekov I, Pardhan S. Temporal ocular coherence tomography-measured changes in anterior chamber angle and diurnal intraocular pressure after laser iridoplasty: IMPACT study. Br J Ophthalmol. 2017;101(7):886–91. https://doi.org/10.1136/bjophthalmol-2016-308720.

40. Bellezza AJ, Hart RT, Burgoyne CF. The optic nerve head as a biomechanical structure: initial finite element modeling. Invest Ophthalmol Vis Sci. 2000;41(10):2991–3000.

41. Burgoyne CF, Downs JC, Bellezza AJ, Suh JK, Hart RT. The optic nerve head as a biomechanical structure: a new paradigm for understanding the role of IOP-related stress and strain in the pathophysiology of glaucomatous optic nerve head damage. Prog Retin Eye Res. 2005;24(1):39–73. https://doi.org/10.1016/j.preteyeres.2004.06.001.

42. Tamm ER, Ethier CR, Lasker/IRRF Initiative on Astrocytes and Glaucomatous Neurodegeneration Participants. Biological aspects of axonal damage in glaucoma: a brief review. Exp Eye Res. 2017;157:5–12. https://doi.org/10.1016/j.exer.2017.02.006.

43. Nouri-Mahdavi K, Hoffman D, Coleman AL, Liu G, Li G, Gaasterland D, Caprioli J, Advanced Glaucoma Intervention Study. Predictive factors for glaucomatous visual field progression in the advanced Glaucoma intervention Study. Ophthalmology. 2004;111(9):1627–35. https://doi.org/10.1016/j.ophtha.2004.02.017.

44. Caprioli J, Coleman AL. Intraocular pressure fluctuation a risk factor for visual field progression at low intraocular pressures in the advanced glaucoma intervention study. Ophthalmology. 2008;115(7):1123–1129.e3. https://doi.org/10.1016/j.ophtha.2007.10.031.

45. Bengtsson B, Leske MC, Hyman L, Heijl A, Early Manifest Glaucoma Trial Group. Fluctuation of intraocular pressure and glaucoma progression in the early manifest glaucoma trial. Ophthalmology. 2007;114(2):205–9. https://doi.org/10.1016/j.ophtha.2006.07.060.

46. Medeiros FA, Weinreb RN, Zangwill LM, Alencar LM, Sample PA, Vasile C, Bowd C. Long-term intraocular pressure fluctuations and risk of conversion from ocular hypertension to glaucoma. Ophthalmology. 2008;115(6):934–40. https://doi.org/10.1016/j.ophtha.2007.08.012.

47. Jonas JB, Budde WM, Stroux A, Oberacher-Velten IM, Jünemann A. Diurnal intraocular pressure profiles and progression of chronic open-angle glaucoma. Eye (Lond). 2007;21(7):948–51. https://doi.org/10.1038/sj.eye.6702351.

48. Guo ZZ, Chang K, Wei X. Intraocular pressure fluctuation and the risk of glaucomatous damage deterioration: a meta-analysis. Int J Ophthalmol. 2019;12(1):123–8. https://doi.org/10.18240/ijo.2019.01.19.

49. Tan S, Yu M, Baig N, Chan PP, Tang FY, Tham CC. Circadian intraocular pressure fluctuation and disease progression in primary angle closure Glaucoma. Invest Ophthalmol Vis Sci. 2015;56(8):4994–5005. https://doi.org/10.1167/iovs.15-17245.

50. Baskaran M, Kumar RS, Govindasamy CV, Htoon HM, Wong CY, Perera SA, Wong TT, Aung T. Diurnal intraocular pressure fluctuation and associated risk factors in eyes with angle closure. Ophthalmology. 2009;116(12):2300–4. https://doi.org/10.1016/j.ophtha.2009.06.010.

51. Chen YY, Sun LP, Thomas R, Liang YB, Fan SJ, Sun X, Li SZ, Zhang SD, Wang NL. Long-term intraocular pressure fluctuation of primary angle closure disease following laser peripheral iridotomy/iridoplasty. Chin Med J. 2011;124(19):3066–9.

52. Arora T, Bali SJ, Arora V, Wadhwani M, Panda A, Dada T. Diurnal versus office-hour intraocular pressure fluctuation in primary adult onset glaucoma. J Opt. 2015;8(4):239–43. https://doi.org/10.1016/j.optom.2014.05.005.

Objective Quantitative Evaluation of Angle Closure

3

Yu Meng Wang and Carol Y. Cheung

Abstract

Several limitations have been encountered with the reference standard of gonioscopy for angle assessment. Advancements in ophthalmic imaging technologies, especially anterior segment optical coherence tomography (AS-OCT) in recent years, have established robust, reliable, and quantitative protocols to examine the structure of the anterior segment with proven usefulness to detect various ocular complications including angle closure. The goal of this chapter is to review the basics of the most commonly used anterior segment imaging techniques (ultrasound biomicroscopy and AS-OCT), including a concise update of how they work and how objective and quantitative evaluation can be conducted in clinical practice.

Keywords

Angle closure · Anterior segment OCT · Anterior segment

Y. M. Wang · C. Y. Cheung (✉)
Department of Ophthalmology and Visual Sciences,
The Chinese University of Hong Kong,
Hong Kong, China
e-mail: carolcheung@cuhk.edu.hk

3.1 Introduction

Angle closure diseases can be classified into different subtypes including primary angle closure suspect (PACS), acute angle closure (AAC), and primary angle closure glaucoma (PACG) [1]. Among them, PACG is potentially blinding, and so far, with no cure. Control of intraocular pressure (IOP) helps inhibition of disease progression in some patients. These subtypes can also represent different stages of disease severities. Individuals who are PACS can advance to AAC, and further to PACG, which is potentially blinding. The advancements are affected by both inductive and constitutive risk factors, while some patients remain stable in their ocular conditions. Several ocular risk factors have been identified for angle closure disease. These include short axial length, shallow anterior chamber (AC), thick peripheral iris roll (PIR), and thick and anteriorly positioned lens [2]. Qualitative and quantitative evaluation of the anterior segment in these eyes are helpful in understanding the pathogenesis of angle closure [3], and thus can provide clues to further disease development. Consequentially, prediction may be possible.

Traditional approaches, such as UBM, for anterior chamber angle (ACA) imaging mostly work on obtaining a single cross-sectional slice view across the anterior segment Furthermore, quantitative analysis of these images requires expertise to conduct the analysis. Interpretations

© Springer Nature Singapore Pte Ltd. 2021
C. C. Y. Tham (ed.), *Primary Angle Closure Glaucoma (PACG)*,
https://doi.org/10.1007/978-981-15-8120-5_3

of the results also need personal experiences and evaluations which, inevitably, can be subjective. Advances in imaging technologies and software in recent years have enhanced the robustness of anterior segment imaging and its quantitative measurement. Newer approaches using swept-source optical coherence tomography (SS-OCT) allow for imaging of the entire ACA over 360 degree and provide a summary measure of the extent of angle closure [4]. Data collection, analysis, and interpretation are aided by high-performance software to obtain objective and quantitative measurements. These modern imaging technologies are expected to be very effectively applied for evaluation of angle closure, especially in long-term management and assessment of disease development [5].

In this chapter, we review the basics of the most commonly used anterior segment imaging techniques (ultrasound biomicroscopy and AS-OCT), including a concise update of how they work and how objective and quantitative evaluation can be conducted in clinical practice.

3.2 Qualitative and Quantitative Evaluation Approaches of the Anterior Segment

3.2.1 Ultrasound Biomicroscopy

Ultrasound Biomicroscopy (UBM) provides highly resolved, reliable, and repeatable images of the anterior segment (Fig. 3.1). Software are available for quantitative measurements, such as ACA, angle opening distance (AOD) and angle recess area (ARA). UBM uses high-frequency ultrasound at 50–100 MHz for anterior segment imaging. A computer program then converts these sound waves into a high-resolution B-scan image. The probe provides a scan rate of 8 Hz and enables a lateral resolution of 50 μm and an axial resolution of 25 μm [6, 7]. UBM has previously been shown to have a good agreement with gonioscopy in its ability to evaluate angle closure when performed in a darkened room [8]. In addition, unlike conventional methodologies of AS-OCT, UBM can achieve visualization of structures posterior to the iris pigment epithelium [6, 7, 9, 10] as sound penetrates the pigment epithelium but light does not. Thus, UBM is capable for visualizing fine details of the posterior chamber structures, including the lens zonules, ciliary body, and even the anterior choroid. Unlike AS-OCT, UBM can also be performed with the subject lying down, and thus it is useful in the operating room when examination is needed for the patient under anesthesia. However, UBM is an eye contact method and requires highly skilled technicians or doctors to operate Table 3.1 highlights the main differences between AS-OCT and UBM. It is noted that prior studies have reported excellent intra-observer reproducibility but poor inter-observer repro-

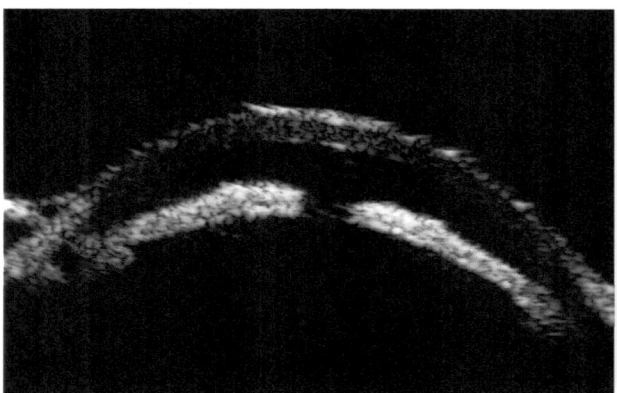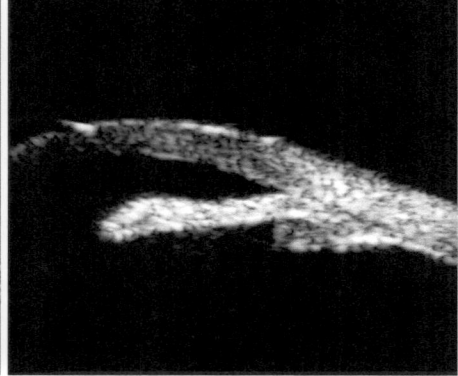

Fig. 3.1 Anterior chamber and its angle imaged by UBM

ducibility in assessing the ACA or iris dimensions measured from UBM images [11, 12]. In addition, UBM may have a narrower field of view compared to the AS-OCT [13–15].

Table 3.1 Comparison of UBM and AS-OCT in anterior segment imaging

UBM	AS-OCT
Require contact and a liquid coupling medium	Noncontact
Mild patient discomfort	No patient discomfort apart from some patience is required during the measurement
Skilled operator requiring experience	Non-skilled operator can be readily trained
Lower axial resolution	High axial resolution
Capable to visualize structures posterior to the iris pigment epithelium	Limited ability to visualize structures posterior to the iris pigment epithelium
Slower acquisition time	Fast acquisition time
Smaller field of view	Wide field of view
Seated upright or supine positions	Seated upright position
Can image through opaque corneas	Use for clear corneas

AS-OCT Anterior segment optical coherence tomography, *UBM* Ultrasound biomicroscopy

3.2.2 Anterior Segment Optical Coherence Tomography

Anterior Segment Optical Coherence Tomography (AS-OCT) is a non-contact and rapid imaging device that uses low-coherence interferometry to obtain cross-sectional images of the anterior segment [16]. Figure 3.2 shows the structure of anterior segment imaged by AS-OCT. Studies have shown that measurements from the cross-sectional AS-OCT images, such as anterior chamber depth (ACD), anterior chamber area, AOD, trabecular iris space area (TISA), and iris thickness, are with good reproducibility [17, 18]. Unlike gonioscopy, the measurement is objective and not operator dependent. There are advanced models of AS-OCT based on different configurations, including time-domain (TD-OCT), spectral-domain (SD-OCT), and swept-source (SS-OCT) [19]. Table 3.2 summarizes the features of each of these configurations. Imaging based on SS-OCT and SD-OCT are considered a type of Fourier-domain (FD) OCT. Compared with TD-OCT, the inherent signal-to-noise ratio is lower and the imaging speed (up to 20–40 kHz line-scan rate) of FD-based OCT is higher.

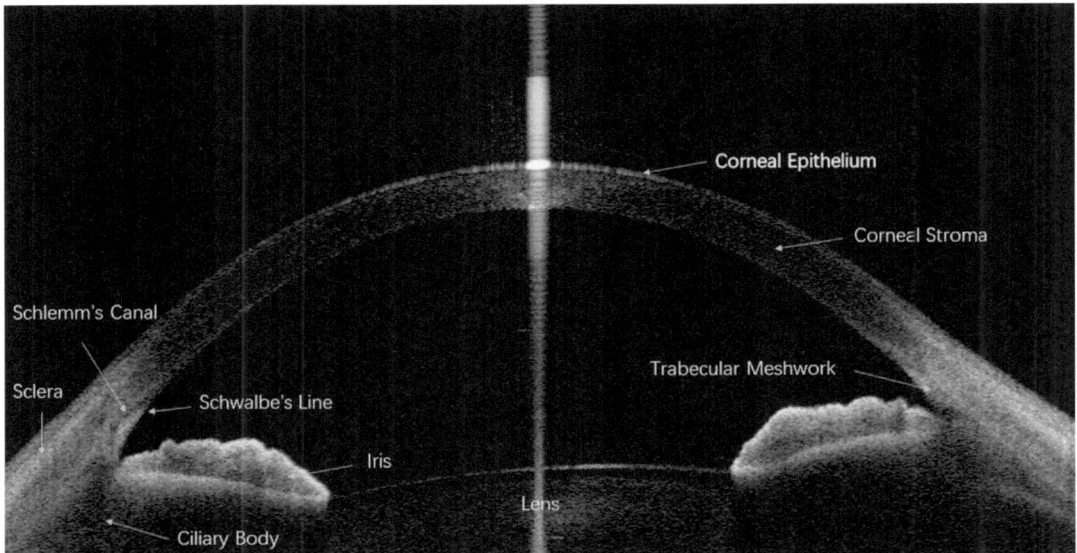

Fig. 3.2 Structure of anterior segment imaged by AS-OCT

Table 3.2 Comparison of different modes of AS-OCT

	Time-domain AS-OCT	Posterior segment spectral-domain OCT	Swept-source AS-OCT
Types	Zeiss Visante, Heidelberg SL-OCT	Spectralis OCT, Cirrus HDOCT, Optovue OCT	Casia SS-1000 OCT Casia2
Central wavelength	1310 nm	880 nm (Spectralis) 840 nm (Cirrus & Optovue)	1310 nm
Axial resolution	>15 μm	<5 μm	10 μm
Imaging depth range	6–7 mm	2–3 mm	6 mm
Line-scan rate	2 kHz/200 HZ	20–40 kHz	30 kHz

AS-OCT Anterior segment optical coherence tomography, *SL-OCT* Slit-lamp optical coherence tomography

With the advent of AS-OCT, imaging researchers can capture the entire cross-section of the anterior segment in a single high-resolution image to enable precise assessment of lens, in addition to the angle and iris parameters. Lens vault (LV), defined as the perpendicular distance between the anterior lens pole and the horizontal line joining the temporal and nasal scleral spurs (SSs), is a structural parameter associated with angle closure that can be measured with AS-OCT [20, 21]. There are reported patients with exaggerated LV in which the iris appeared to drape the anterior surface of the lens, giving rise to a "volcano-like configuration" without an increase in iris curvature (I-curve) [17]. As the I-curve has been reported to be only moderately correlated with increased LV, pupil block may not be the only mechanism by which increased LV causes angle closure [22].

Shabana et al. assessed four different mechanisms of primary angle closure (PAC) by evaluating AS-OCT images: pupil block, plateau iris configuration, thick peripheral iris roll (PIR), and exaggerated LV. They reported significant differences in quantitative angle closure parameters for these different PAC mechanisms. This classification scheme may be effective for the evaluation of progression of individuals with angle closure into angle diseases [17].

3.2.2.1 Posterior Segment Spectral-Domain OCT

With the use of an external adaptor lens, posterior segment Segment Spectral-Domain OCT (SD-OCT) such as Spectralis OCT, Cirrus HDOCT, and Optovue OCT, is also possible to image the anterior chamber of an eye [23–25]. The Spectralis uses shorter 880 nm wavelength light to produce higher axial-resolution images, which permits visualization of intraocular structures such as Schwalbe's line and Schlemm's canal [26, 27]. However, the shorter wavelength also results in a shorter imaging range, thus precluding visualization of the entire anterior chamber in a single scan. Previous study identified good intra-device reproducibility and good inter-device agreement of anterior segment parameter measurement values for the CASIA2 and Spectralis OCT2 [25].

3.2.2.2 Swept-Source OCT

Swept-Source OCT (SS-OCT) is the latest generation of OCT and is currently commercially available. It utilizes a swept-source laser wavelength of 1310 nm based on FD technology and employing a scan speed of 30,000 A-scans/second and an axial resolution of 10 μm. Such capabilities enable capturing images of extremely high resolution. One commonly used model is the Casia SS-1000 OCT (Tomey, Nagoya, Japan). Less than 3 seconds are needed to image the angle morphology in high-resolution and circumferentially 360°. Examples of eyes with open angle and closed angle were shown in Figs. 3.3, 3.4, 3.5 and 3.6.

3.2.2.3 Comparison Between UBM and AS-OCT

Compared with UBM, AS-OCT achieves better resolution and does not require contact with the

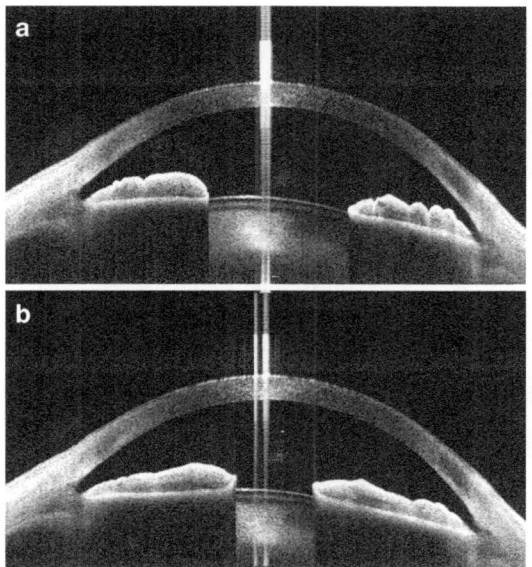

Fig. 3.3 Example of open angle in cross-sectional view: (**a**) imaged in dark condition; (**b**) Imaged in lighting condition

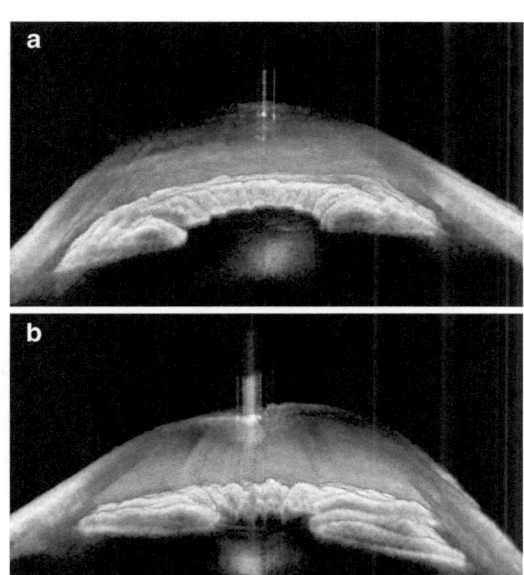

Fig. 3.5 Example of open angle in 3D view: (**a**) imaged in dark condition; (**b**) imaged in lighting condition

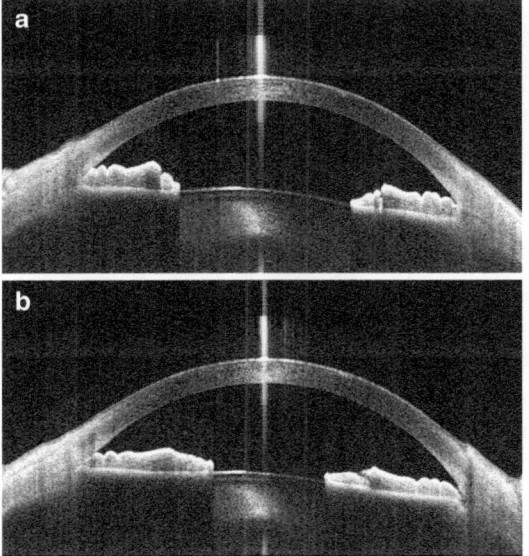

Fig. 3.4 Example of closed angle in cross-sectional view: (**a**) imaged in dark; (**b**) imaged in lighting condition

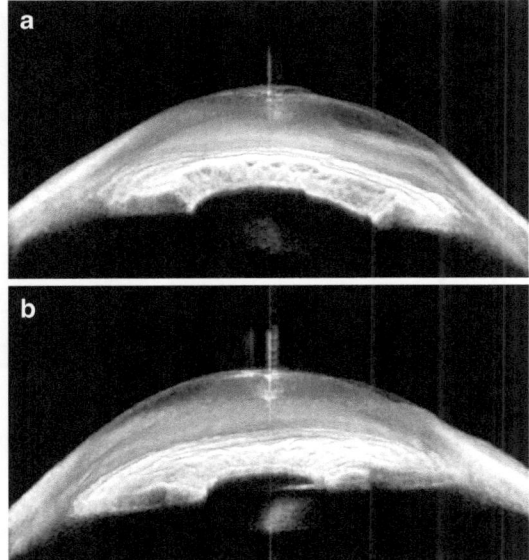

Fig. 3.6 Example of closed angle in 3D view: (**a**) imaged in dark condition; (**b**) imaged in lighting condition

ocular surface [28]. The main limitation of AS-OCT is that the light energy cannot penetrate tissues behind the iris pigment epithelium. Consequently, AS-OCT cannot visualize any structures posterior to the iris pigment epithelium. Thus, AS-OCT is not useful in the detection of ocular complications such as plateau iris syndrome and phacomorphic angle-closure (Table 3.1).

3.3   Quantitative Metrics of Angle Closure

3.3.1   Quantitative Metrics in 2D AS-OCT Images

Biometric analysis of the ACA requires a reference landmark from which the angle measurements are derived. Typically, the scleral spur (SS) (Fig. 3.7) is used as a reference point for structural measurements of AOD, [9] TISA, ARA, [29] scleral thickness, [11] trabecular meshwork-ciliary process distance, and [11] trabecular iris angle (TIA) [9, 15] (Fig. 3.8). Other biometric parameters that can be measured by the AS-OCT include iris thickness, iris curvature, AC depth, AC width, and lens vault [30]. These parameters are further described in Table 3.3. Although these

AS-OCT parameters, including ACD and ACA, [22] have been shown to differ in various subtypes of angle closure disease, characteristic features that may predict development to PACG from eyes with narrow angles have not yet been established.

Manual identification of the SS prior to measurements is important to the accuracy of the measurements of various biometric parameters. But there are disadvantages in the use of SS as an anchor for high-resolution imaging [11]. There is currently no technology available that can automatically identify the SS. Difficulty in identifying the SS as a reference point has been cited in numerous studies, with reportedly 15–28% of AS-OCT images not able to identify the SS [31, 32]. So far, there is no consensus regarding the relationships between various AS-OCT obtained

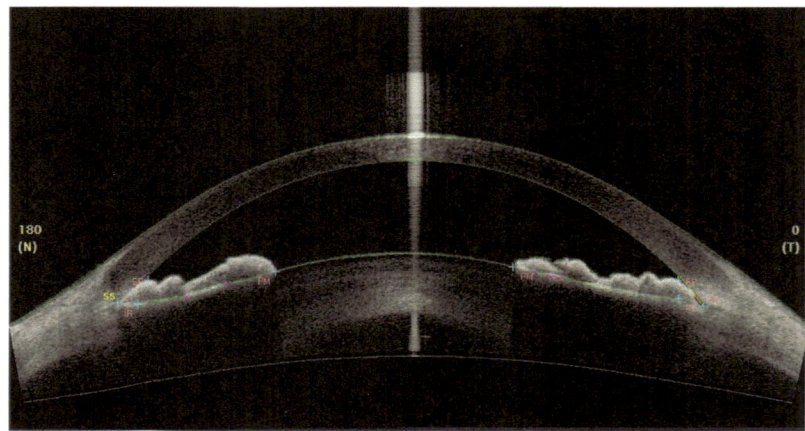

Fig. 3.7 Landmarks of anterior segment structure for quantitative measurement of ACA: Scleral Spur (SS), ITC End Point (EP), and Iris Root (IR)

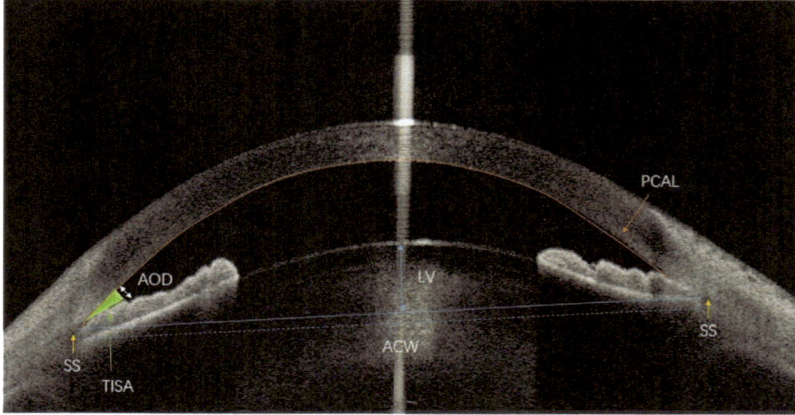

Fig. 3.8 Measurement of anterior segment parameters on a cross-sectional anterior segment optical coherence tomography image. *ACW* anterior chamber width, *AOD* anterior opening distance, *SS* scleral spur, *LV* lens vault, *PCAL* posterior corneal arc length, *TISA* trabecular iris space area

Table 3.3 Definitions of quantitative AS-OCT biometric parameters

Parameter	Group	Abbreviation	Unit	Description
Angle opening distance	ACA related	AOD	μm	Linear distance between the point of the inner corneoscleral wall and the iris
Angle recess area	ACA related	ARA	μm²	The triangular area demarcated by the anterior iris surface, corneal endothelium, and a line perpendicular to the corneal endothelium drawn from a point 750 μm anterior to the scleral spur to the iris surface
Trabecular iris angle	ACA related	TIA	Degree	Angle formed from angle recess to points 500 μm from scleral spur on trabecular meshwork and perpendicular on surface of iris
Trabecular iris space area	ACA related	TISA	mm²	A trapezoidal area measuring the filtering area. The defining boundaries for this trapezoidal area are: Anteriorly, the AOD; posteriorly, a line drawn from the scleral spur perpendicular to the plane of the inner scleral wall to the opposing iris; superiorly, the inner corneoscleral wall; and inferiorly, the iris surface
Iris thickness	Iris related	IT	mm	Measured from a perpendicular point 500 μm or 750 μm from the scleral spur, with the scleral spur defined as the point at which a change in the curvature of the inner surface of the angle is apparent
Iris cross-sectional area	Iris related	IA	mm²	The average of the cross-sectional area of both nasal and temporal and nasal sides
Iris curvature	Iris related	IC	mm	Maximum perpendicular distance between iris pigment epithelium and line, connecting the most peripheral to most central point of the epithelium
Iris–trabecular contact index	Iris related	ITC index	NA	The ITC index was calculated as a percentage of the angle that was closed on SSOCT images. The ITC graph with the Y-axis representing ITC and the X-axis representing the degree of the angle. The graph above the red horizontal line demonstrates the amount of angle closure measured as the ITC index in percentage
Anterior chamber depth	AC related	ACD	mm	Distance from corneal endothelium to anterior surface of the lens
Anterior chamber width	AC related	ACW	mm	Distance of a horizontal line joining the two scleral spurs
Anterior chamber volume	AC related	ACV	mm³	The volume of anterior chamber
Lens vault	Lens related	LV	mm	Perpendicular distance between anterior pole of the crystalline lens and the horizontal line joining the two scleral spurs
Scleral thickness	NA	ST	mm	Measured perpendicular from the scleral spur to the episcleral surface

AS-OCT Anterior segment optical coherence tomography, *AC* Anterior chamber, *ACA* Anterior chamber angle

parameters and the aqueous humor outflow. According to a recent study, Spectralis OCT with enhanced depth imaging (EDI) is able to reveal detailed optic nerve head features and different laminar and prelaminar EDI OCT-derived parameters can be obtained to characterize glaucomatous features [33]. A previous study by Spectralis OCT with EDI had identified the Schwalbe's line and scleral spur in all nasal and temporal scans [34]. In another study, by Cheung et al., using a modified Cirrus SD-OCT, the Schwalbe's line (Fig. 3.9) was identifiable in 95% of the scans and the SS was identifiable in 85% of glaucoma patients [26]. In the Casia OCT, the SS was identifiable in all study subjects. However, Schlemm's canal was only identifiable in 32% of the scans.

Fig. 3.9 The Schwalbe's line was identifiable in 95% of the scans and the scleral spur was identifiable in 85% of glaucoma patients

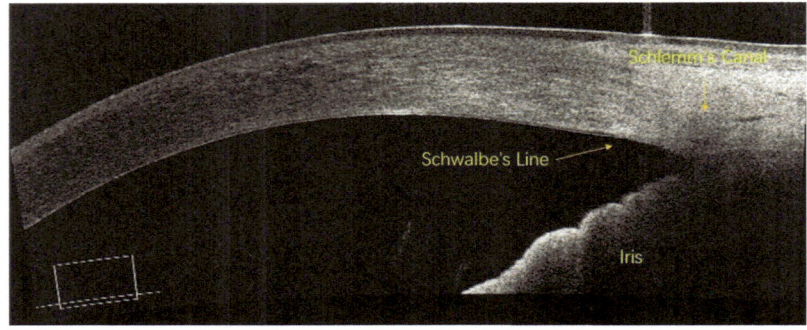

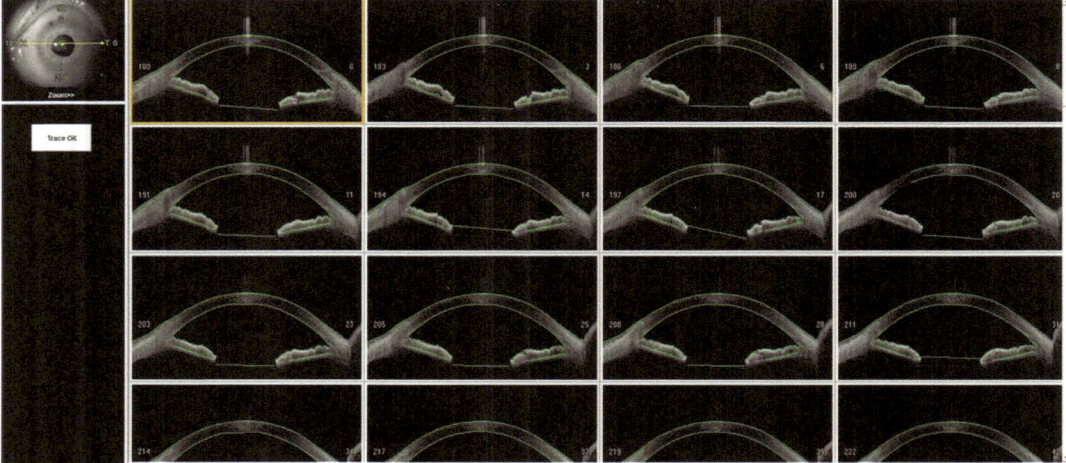

Fig. 3.10 Measurement of iris volume and anterior chamber volume with SS-OCT (This screenshot shows part of the scanning)

Its identification has also been previously reported to be subject to measurement error and variability [11, 35–37]. Accurate identification of the SS is hampered by various ocular features or conditions such as eye quadrant [31], small AC depth, narrow angle, short axial length, and older age [38]. But accurate identification of the position of the SS using AS-OCT is very important. There are many reported attempts to improve the techniques as to best identify the SS. The three most common technical approaches are (1) location of Schwalbe's line relative to the scleral spur, (2) the intersection of the ciliary muscle (CM) and the inner corneal margin, and (3) a bump-like structure in the inner corneal-meshwork margin. A study by Seager et al. demonstrated that among these three different methods, the CM approach demonstrated the highest rate of scleral spur identification with the lowest intra- and inter-observer variability [39].

Besides, the dynamic dark-light changes of the anterior chamber angle can be captured with real-time video recording and analyzed with anterior segment OCT [40]. Previous study identified that the angle width generally decreased linearly with increasing pupil diameter, and the differences of the angle width measured in the dark and in the light varied substantially among individuals [40].

3.3.2 Quantitative Metrics in 3D AS-OCT Images

The SS-OCT's low-density 3-dimensional angle analysis scan simultaneously obtains multiple radial scans of the whole anterior chamber for the entire circumference of the angle. The instrument software automatically detected the anterior and posterior boundaries of the iris and cornea in the individual B-scans (Fig. 3.10) [41]. The iris root was defined as the intersection of the anterior and posterior iris boundaries and the ciliary body. The anterior iris boundary was detected as the anterior chamber, anterior iris surface interface, whereas the posterior iris boundary was detected as the external border of the iris pigment epithe-

lium. The iris volume was calculated as a summation of pixel volume derived from individual B-scans [41]. In-built software analysis then analyzes the extent of iris–trabecular contact (ITC) across 360° of the angle and calculates the extent of angle-closure as the ITC index [42]. The examples of ITC index calculation were shown in Fig. 3.11. In addition, SS-OCT allows visualization and reproducible measurements of the area and degree of peripheral anterior synechia (PAS) involvement (Fig. 3.12), providing a

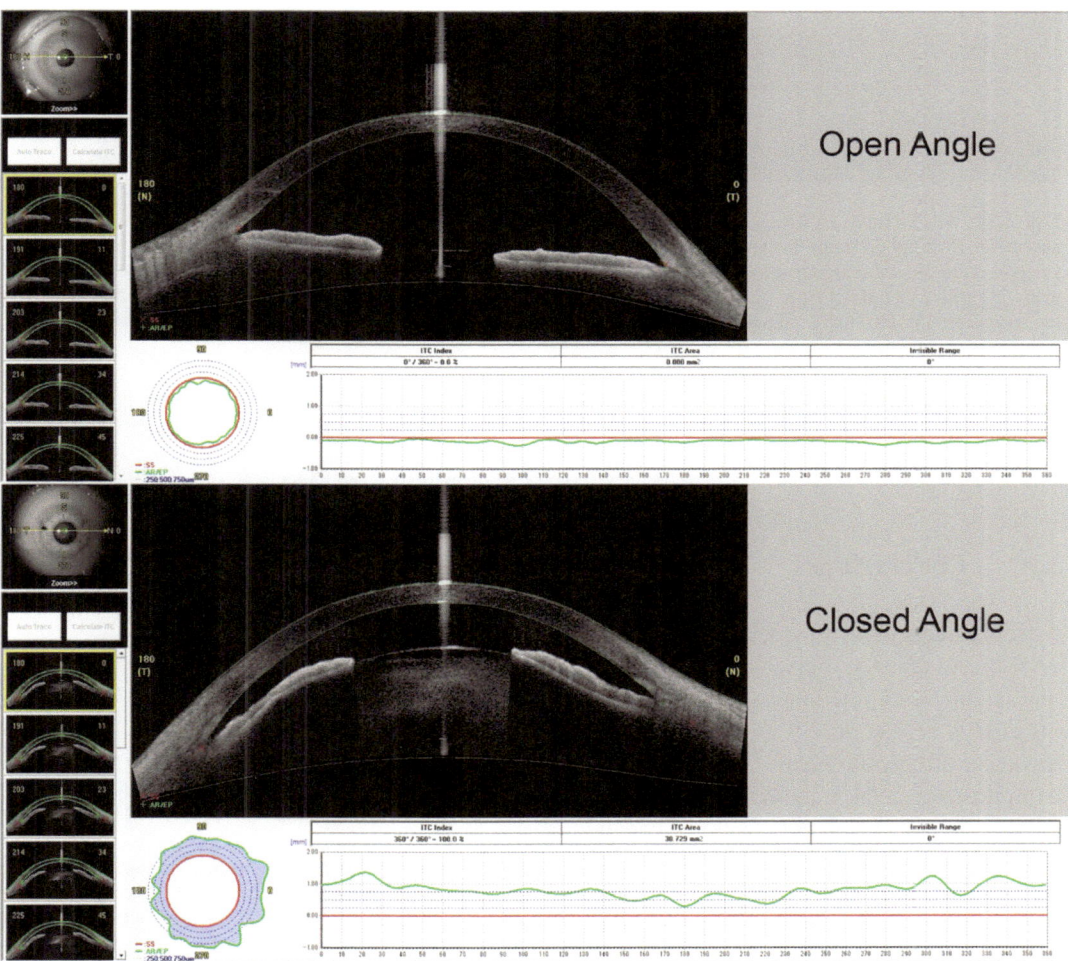

Fig. 3.11 The iridotrabecular contact (ITC) index analysis for open angle and closed angle. The "x" represents the scleral spur (SS) markings and the "+" represents the ITC end-point (EP). Both points are marked by an observer grading the image. The ITC chart with the blue area representing the amount and distribution of ITC. The dashed lines indicate 250 μm, 500 μm, and 750 μm from the scleral spur. The ITC graph with the Y-axis representing ITC (in arbitrary units) and the X-axis representing the degree of the angle. The graph above the red horizontal line (representing SS) demonstrates the amount of angle-closure measured as the ITC index in percentage (in red oval circle)

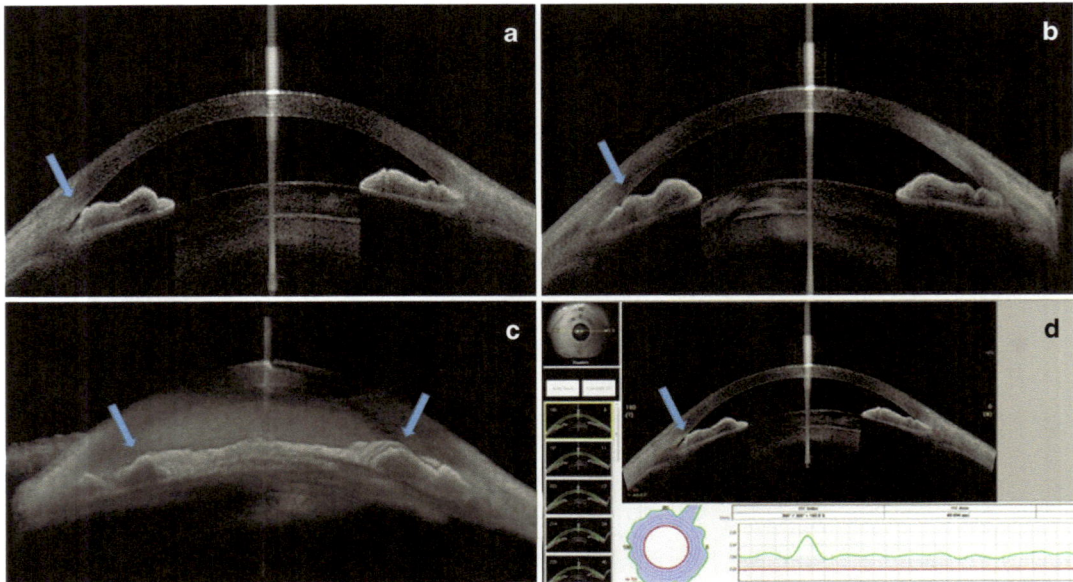

Fig. 3.12 An example showing the imaging and measurement of peripheral anterior synechia (PAS) with the swept-source optical coherence tomography (OCT) in an eye with primary angle-closure glaucoma. The horizontal (**a**) and vertical (**b**) OCT images are shown. Three-dimensional reconstruction of the OCT images reveals PAS (**c**). A polar plot of the PAS is shown in (**d**), with the red line representing the location of the scleral spur and the green line representing the location of the anterior tip of the irido-angle adhesion

new paradigm for evaluation of PAS progression and risk assessment for development of angle-closure glaucoma [43].

3.4   Conclusions

Advancements in imaging technologies and software have allowed objective and quantitative measurements of fine inner structures of the retina at high resolution. SS-OCT, with other OCT modes, efficiently and effectively detect complicated retinal features of individuals with angle closure. Computerization capabilities enable standardized procedure in collecting investigative data from individuals for objective and quantitative analysis. These current technologies can fully utilized to study a large number of individuals with angle closure, angle closure diseases such as PACG, and to follow them longitudinally to reveal their disease development [5]. Such information will provide data for biomarkers of PACG development.

Acknowledgments Prof. Clement C. Tham, Dr. Poemen Chan, and Ms. Annie Ling from the Department of Ophthalmology and Visual Sciences, The Chinese University of Hong Kong.

Compliance with Ethical Requirements Carol Y. Cheung and Yu Meng Wang declare that they have no conflict of interest. No human or animal studies were performed by the authors for this article.

References

1. Foster PJ, Buhrmann R, Quigley HA, Johnson GJ. The definition and classification of glaucoma in prevalence surveys. Br J Ophthalmol. 2002;86:238–42.
2. George R, et al. Ocular biometry in occludable angles and angle closure glaucoma: a population based survey. Br J Ophthalmol. 2003;87:399–402.
3. Liu L. Deconstructing the mechanisms of angle closure with anterior segment optical coherence tomography. Clin Exp Ophthalmol. 2011;39:614–22. https://doi.org/10.1111/j.1442-9071.2011.02521.x.
4. Wylegala E, Teper S, Nowinska AK, Milka M, Dobrowolski D. Anterior segment imaging: fourier-domain optical coherence tomography versus time-domain optical coherence tomography. J

Cataract Refract Surg. 2009;35:1410–4. https://doi.org/10.1016/j.jcrs.2009.03.034.

5. Cheung CY, et al. Factors associated with long-term intraocular pressure fluctuation in primary angle closure disease: the CUHK PACG longitudinal (CUPAL) study. J Glaucoma. 2018;27:703–10. https://doi.org/10.1097/IJG.0000000000000996.

6. Pavlin CJ, Harasiewicz K, Sherar MD, Foster FS. Clinical use of ultrasound biomicroscopy. Ophthalmology. 1991;98:287–95.

7. Pavlin CJ, Sherar MD, Foster FS. Subsurface ultrasound microscopic imaging of the intact eye. Ophthalmology. 1990;97:244–50.

8. Barkana Y, Dorairaj SK, Gerber Y, Liebmann JM, Ritch R. Agreement between gonioscopy and ultrasound biomicroscopy in detecting iridotrabecular apposition. Arch Ophthalmol. 2007;125:1331–5. https://doi.org/10.1001/archopht.125.10.1331.

9. Pavlin CJ, Harasiewicz K, Foster FS. Ultrasound biomicroscopy of anterior segment structures in normal and glaucomatous eyes. Am J Ophthalmol. 1992;113:381–9.

10. Urbak SF, Pedersen JK, Thorsen TT. Ultrasound biomicroscopy. II. Intraobserver and interobserver reproducibility of measurements. Acta Ophthalmol Scand. 1998;76:546–9.

11. Tello C, Liebmann J, Potash SD, Cohen H, Ritch R. Measurement of ultrasound biomicroscopy images: intraobserver and interobserver reliability. Invest Ophthalmol Vis Sci. 1994;35:3549–52.

12. Zhang Q, Jin W, Wang Q. Repeatability, reproducibility, and agreement of central anterior chamber depth measurements in pseudophakic and phakic eyes: optical coherence tomography versus ultrasound biomicroscopy. J Cataract Refract Surg. 2010;36:941–6. https://doi.org/10.1016/j.jcrs.2009.12.038.

13. Dada T, Sihota R, Gadia R, Aggarwal A, Mandal S, Gupta V. Comparison of anterior segment optical coherence tomography and ultrasound biomicroscopy for assessment of the anterior segment. J Cataract Refract Surg. 2007;33:837–40. https://doi.org/10.1016/j.jcrs.2007.01.021.

14. Memarzadeh F, Li Y, Chopra V, Varma R, Francis BA, Huang D. Anterior segment optical coherence tomography for imaging the anterior chamber after laser peripheral iridotomy. Am J Ophthalmol. 2007;143:877–9. https://doi.org/10.1016/j.ajo.2006.11.055.

15. Radhakrishnan S, et al. Comparison of optical coherence tomography and ultrasound biomicroscopy for detection of narrow anterior chamber angles. Arch Ophthalmol. 2005;123:1053–9. https://doi.org/10.1001/archopht.123.8.1053.

16. Radhakrishnan S, Rollins AM, Roth JE, Yazdanfar S, Westphal V, Bardenstein DS, Izatt JA. Real-time optical coherence tomography of the anterior segment at 1310 nm. Arch Ophthalmol. 2001;119:1179–85.

17. Shabana N, et al. Quantitative evaluation of anterior chamber parameters using anterior segment optical coherence tomography in primary angle closure mechanisms. Clin Exp Ophthalmol. 2012;40:792–801. https://doi.org/10.1111/j.1442-9071.2012.02805.x.

18. Sng CC, et al. Determinants of anterior chamber depth: the Singapore Chinese eye study. Ophthalmology. 2012;119:1143–50. https://doi.org/10.1016/j.ophtha.2012.01.011.

19. Li P, Johnstone M, Wang RK. Full anterior segment biometry with extended imaging range spectral domain optical coherence tomography at 1340 nm. J Biomed Opt. 2014;19:046013. https://doi.org/10.1117/1.JBO.19.4.046013.

20. Nongpiur ME, et al. Lens vault, thickness, and position in Chinese subjects with angle closure. Ophthalmology. 2011;118:474–9. https://doi.org/10.1016/j.ophtha.2010.07.025.

21. Nongpiur ME, et al. Novel association of smaller anterior chamber width with angle closure in Singaporeans. Ophthalmology. 2010;117:1967–73. https://doi.org/10.1016/j.ophtha.2010.02.007.

22. Moghimi S, et al. Ocular biometry in the subtypes of angle closure: an anterior segment optical coherence tomography study. Am J Ophthalmol. 2013;155:664–673, 673 e661. https://doi.org/10.1016/j.ajo.2012.10.014.

23. Ramos JL, Li Y, Huang D. Clinical and research applications of anterior segment optical coherence tomography – a review. Clin Exp Ophthalmol. 2009;37:81–9. https://doi.org/10.1111/j.1442-9071 2008.01823.x.

24. Rodrigues EB, Johanson M, Penha FM. Anterior segment tomography with the cirrus optical coherence tomography. J Ophthalmol. 2012;2012:806989. https://doi.org/10.1155/2012/806989.

25. Xu BY, Mai DD, Penteado RC, Saunders L, Weinreb RN. Reproducibility and agreement of anterior segment parameter measurements obtained using the CASIA2 and Spectralis OCT2 optical coherence tomography devices. J Glaucoma. 2017;26:974–9. https://doi.org/10.1097/IJG.0000000000000788.

26. Cheung CY, et al. Novel anterior-chamber angle measurements by high-definition optical coherence tomography using the Schwalbe line as the landmark. Br J Ophthalmol. 2011;95:955–9. https://doi.org/10.1136/bjo.2010.189217.

27. Kagemann L, et al. Identification and assessment of Schlemm's canal by spectral-domain optical coherence tomography. Invest Ophthalmol Vis Sci. 2010;51:4054–9. https://doi.org/10.1167/iovs.09-4559.

28. Fukuda S, Kawana K, Yasuno Y, Oshika T. Repeatability and reproducibility of anterior chamber volume measurements using 3-dimensional corneal and anterior segment optical coherence tomography. J Cataract Refract Surg. 2011;37:461–8. https://doi.org/10.1016/j.jcrs.2010.08.053.

29. Ishikawa H, Esaki K, Liebmann JM, Uji Y, Ritch R. Ultrasound biomicroscopy dark room provocative testing: a quantitative method for estimating anterior chamber angle width. Jpn J Ophthalmol. 1999;43:526–34.

30. Sung KR, Lee KS, Hong JW. Baseline anterior segment parameters associated with the long-term outcome of laser peripheral Iridotomy. Curr Eye Res. 2015;40:1128–33. https://doi.org/10.3109/02713683.2014.986334.

31. Sakata LM, Lavanya R, Friedman DS, Aung HT, Seah SK, Foster PJ, Aung T. Assessment of the scleral spur in anterior segment optical coherence tomography images. Arch Ophthalmol. 2008b;126:181–5. https://doi.org/10.1001/archophthalmol.2007.46.

32. Wang BS, et al. Increased iris thickness and association with primary angle closure glaucoma. Br J Ophthalmol. 2011;95:46–50. https://doi.org/10.1136/bjo.2009.178129.

33. Lopes FS, Matsubara I, Almeida I, Dorairaj SK, Vessani RM, Paranhos A Jr, Prata TS. Structure-function relationships in glaucoma using enhanced depth imaging optical coherence tomography-derived parameters: a cross-sectional observational study. BMC Ophthalmol. 2019;19:52. https://doi.org/10.1186/s12886-019-1054-9.

34. Day AC, et al. Spectral domain optical coherence tomography imaging of the aqueous outflow structures in normal participants of the EPIC-Norfolk eye study. Br J Ophthalmol. 2013;97:189–95. https://doi.org/10.1136/bjophthalmol-2012-302147.

35. Leung CK, et al. Novel approach for anterior chamber angle analysis: anterior chamber angle detection with edge measurement and identification algorithm (ACADEMIA). Arch Ophthalmol. 2006;124:1395–401. https://doi.org/10.1001/archopht.124.10.1395.

36. Li H, Leung CK, Cheung CY, Wong L, Pang CP, Weinreb RN, Lam DS. Repeatability and reproducibility of anterior chamber angle measurement with anterior segment optical coherence tomography. Br J Ophthalmol. 2007;91:1490–2. https://doi.org/10.1136/bjo.2007.118901.

37. Sakata LM, et al. Comparison of gonioscopy and anterior segment ocular coherence tomography in detecting angle closure in different quadrants of the anterior chamber angle. Ophthalmology. 2008a;115:769–74. https://doi.org/10.1016/j.ophtha.2007.06.030.

38. Liu S, et al. Assessment of scleral spur visibility with anterior segment optical coherence tomography. J Glaucoma. 2010;19:132–5. https://doi.org/10.1097/IJG.0b013e3181a98ce4.

39. Seager FE, Wang J, Arora KS, Quigley HA. The effect of scleral spur identification methods on structural measurements by anterior segment optical coherence tomography. J Glaucoma. 2014;23:e29–38. https://doi.org/10.1097/IJG.0b013e31829e55ae.

40. Leung CK, et al. Dynamic analysis of dark-light changes of the anterior chamber angle with anterior segment OCT. Invest Ophthalmol Vis Sci. 2007;48:4116–22. https://doi.org/10.1167/iovs.07-0010.

41. Mak H, Xu G, Leung CK. Imaging the iris with swept-source optical coherence tomography: relationship between iris volume and primary angle closure. Ophthalmology. 2013;120:2517–24. https://doi.org/10.1016/j.ophtha.2013.05.009.

42. Baskaran M, Ho SW, Tun TA, How AC, Perera SA, Friedman DS, Aung T. Assessment of circumferential angle-closure by the iris-trabecular contact index with swept-source optical coherence tomography. Ophthalmology. 2013;120:2226–31. https://doi.org/10.1016/j.ophtha.2013.04.020.

43. Lai I, Mak H, Lai G, Yu M, Lam DS, Leung CK. Anterior chamber angle imaging with swept-source optical coherence tomography: measuring peripheral anterior synechia in glaucoma. Ophthalmology. 2013;120:1144–9. https://doi.org/10.1016/j.ophtha.2012.12.006.

Medical Therapy in Angle Closure Glaucoma

4

Prin Rojanapongpun and Visanee Tantisevi

Abstract

Medical therapy plays essential roles in the management of angle closure glaucoma (ACG) both in intraocular pressure (IOP) reduction and in modifying angle anatomy. The administration of multiple topical and systemic hypotensive agents usually enable IOP reduction rapidly. Miotics help to prepare the iris for a definitive laser iridotomy or iridoplasty. Anti-inflammatory and analgesic medications must also be employed to reduce associated symptoms. The use of miotics must be cautious as it may worsen angle closure mechanisms like ciliary block and lens-related mechanism. For chronic ACG, medical treatment could be a mainstay if IOP remains persistently high after laser or surgical treatment. All anti-hypertensive agents work with variable effects depending on the stage and mechanism of angle closure. The relevant mode of action, efficacy, and side effect of each different class of hypotensive medications are described in detail. Prostaglandins are the most effective topical hypotensive agent and could reduce IOP in variable degrees of angle closure. New medications and molecules, still novel for ACG, could have potential use in the future.

Keywords

Medical therapy · Hypotensive medications · Angle closure · Glaucoma · Glaucoma medications · IOP lowering mechanism · Effectiveness · Side effect

Medical treatment plays an essential role in various stages in angle closure glaucoma therapy. One must understand that angle closure glaucoma consists of 2 pathologic mechanisms, angle closure, and glaucomatous optic neuropathy. Thus, medical therapy is involved in both modifying the anatomic and physiologic mechanisms of angle closure as well as preventing damage of the retinal ganglion cells and their axons, which are the retinal nerve fibers. In essence, the roles of medical therapy in primary angle closure glaucoma are:

1. Reverse or eliminate angle closure process
2. Control intraocular pressure (IOP) elevation
3. Neuroprotection and neuroregeneration

4.1 Medical Therapy in Modifying Angle Closure Process

As a rule, angle closure mechanisms must be treated or corrected with laser or surgery. There is a definite role of medical therapy depending on what

P. Rojanapongpun (✉) · V. Tantisevi
Glaucoma Research Unit, Department of Ophthalmology, Faculty of Medicine, Chulalongkorn University and King Chulalongkorn Memorial Hospital, Bangkok, Thailand

stage and which mechanism of angle closure are. In general, laser peripheral iridotomy (LPI) is usually attempted as one of the commonest procedures because LPI can reverse the pupillary block component. Pupillary block is the most common mechanism in angle closure glaucoma. Most of the time, LPI prevents recurrence of the acute attack and prevent the progression to chronic angle closure glaucoma if performed early enough. However, following iridotomy, persistent elevations of IOP may occur. It is common that there are multiple angle closure mechanisms other than a pupillary block. These include plateau iris syndrome, crowding of angle, lens component, and ciliary block. Medication can be used to modify the shape of the iris as in plateau iris configuration. Medication can also affect the rotation of the ciliary processes, which may change the lens position. According to the Asia Pacific Glaucoma guidelines, further management after successful angle modification depends on the optic disc and visual field status, and medical treatment is suitable in conjunction with laser PI or other angle modifying modalities, for example, cataract extraction [1].

4.2 Medical Treatment in Acute Angle Closure

In Acute Angle Closure (AAC), IOP rises rapidly, and the patients usually suffer from severe symptoms. The main purpose of medical therapy is to lower IOP as quickly as possible. When the cornea clears enough due to IOP reduction, laser iridotomy or iridoplasty can be performed, and the attack can be broken. The sooner the IOP reduction, the lesser the damage to the iris microstructures and the ganglion cells.

Systemic medications have a very rapid onset and powerful IOP reduction. Oral glycerol and acetazolamide are the agents usually used. If the patients have vomiting, the intravenous route (mannitol or IV acetazolamide) should be considered. The dosage will be described in detail in the dedicated sector of each medication.

Topical drugs, ß-blockers or alpha$_2$-agonists, act as adjuvants to decrease IOP. Pilocarpine is effective when ischemia of iris sphincter is elimi-

nated by the reduction of IOP to a low safe level [2]. In cases where medical therapy fails, laser iridoplasty is an excellent alternative. It has been shown that iridoplasty can modify the angle morphology, increase the angle width, and change iris curvature more effectively than medical treatment. However, mean IOP reduction was not statistically different [3]. Earlier study also found that there were no statistically significant differences in mean IOP and requirement for long-term glaucoma drugs between eyes treated with iridoplasty and systemic medications [4]. A meta-analysis study confirmed higher effectiveness of IOP lowering efficacy at 2 hour with laser iridoplasty but no statistically significant difference was shown for IOP reduction in comparison between iridoplasty and medical treatment at 24 hour [5].

4.3 Medical Treatment in Chronic Angle Closure Glaucoma

Chronic angle closure glaucoma (CACG) can develop after acute or intermittent angle closure, as well as chronic onset that leads to angle closure and chronic IOP rise. As stated earlier, all angle closure eyes must be treated with laser or surgery to modify the angle anatomy. But medical treatment has both mainstay and adjunctive role in IOP control and modifying angle anatomy because laser treatment or surgery alone may fail to bring IOP to a target level. The reason is that most patients with CACG usually present to the clinics quite late, and a significant number of patients have mixed mechanisms of angle closure. Especially in the Asian population, we found that about 30% of CACG eyes with a patent LPI had plateau iris when using ultrasound biomicroscopy to study angle anatomy [6]. This explains why many CACG eyes will need medication or further intervention to control IOP. In essence, treatment for CACG after eliminating the pupillary block or other angle closure mechanisms mostly depends on lowering IOP to prevent pressure-induced optic nerve damage and is similar to the treatment of primary open-angle glaucoma.

Table 4.1 Glaucoma medication classes and their IOP lowering mechanisms

Glaucoma medication classes	Mechanism of IOP reduction		
	⇓ Aqueous production	⇑ TM outflow	⇑ Uveoscleral Outflow
Pilocarpine		√	
Beta-blockers	√		
CAI	√		
Selective alpha-2 agonists	√		√
Prostaglandins analogue			√
ROCK inhibitors		√	
NO-donating agents Latanoprostene bunod (LBN)		√	√
Nipradilol (α1,β adrenergic antagonists)	√		√

4.4 Pharmacologic Agents for Angle Closure

The role of medications in primary angle closure includes:

1. Initial lowering of IOP to facilitate in performing LPI or iridoplasty.
2. Controlling persistent IOP elevation after laser or surgical treatment.
3. Modifying angle and iris configuration.

Parasympathomimetic like pilocarpine is used to constrict pupil, thus stretching and thinning the peripheral iris to facilitate penetration when performing LPI. For laser iridoplasty, pilocarpine help contracting and stretching iris so that contraction burns can be made in the far periphery location of the iris. In term of controlling the IOP, medical treatment act similarly like in open angle glaucoma with additional concern on the action that affecting angle configuration or iris contour. These actions could result in more or less favorable IOP control based on the mechanism of angle closure. For example, pilocarpine help open up the angle in plateau iris syndrome but can lead to anterior chamber shallowing and narrowing of angle in ciliary block or ciliary congestion.

There are varieties of IOP lowering drugs: topical ß-blocker, prostaglandins, alpha-agonist, miotics, systemic (oral/intravenous) and topical carbonic anhydrase inhibitor, oral hyperosmotic agent, and intravenous hyperosmotic agent. The mechanism of IOP reduction is summarized in Table 4.1 and the site of action (Fig. 4.1). Topical steroids may also be used to control inflammation.

4.4.1 Topical ß-Blocker

Topical ß-blockers lower IOP by reducing aqueous production, most likely through the inhibition of catecholamine-stimulated synthesis of c-AMP in the ciliary epithelium. They are the most commonly prescribed for treatment of both open and angle closure glaucoma in most parts of the world, including Asia.

Timolol, a nonselective ß-blocker, reduces IOP by 20–30% on average. It is most effective during waking hours, but has little effect on aqueous humor production during sleep [7]. The IOP lowering effect peaks at 2 hour after administration and lasts for 24 hours. All nonselective ß-blockers have quite similar hypotensive efficacy. However, different agents and preparation may have slightly different local side effects.

We studied 500 eyes at the ophthalmology clinic in Chulalongkorn hospital (unpublished data) by instilling different preparation of ß-blockers in a random fashion. We assessed and compared ocular comfort and stinging sensation by using a balanced salt solution as a control. We found that carteolol seems to have a favorable ocular tolerability profile when compared with other topical beta-blockers. The level of comfort or the degree of irritation is similar to the control BSS. Betaxolol (as Betoptic-S™), timolol, and levobunolol are almost equally comfortable

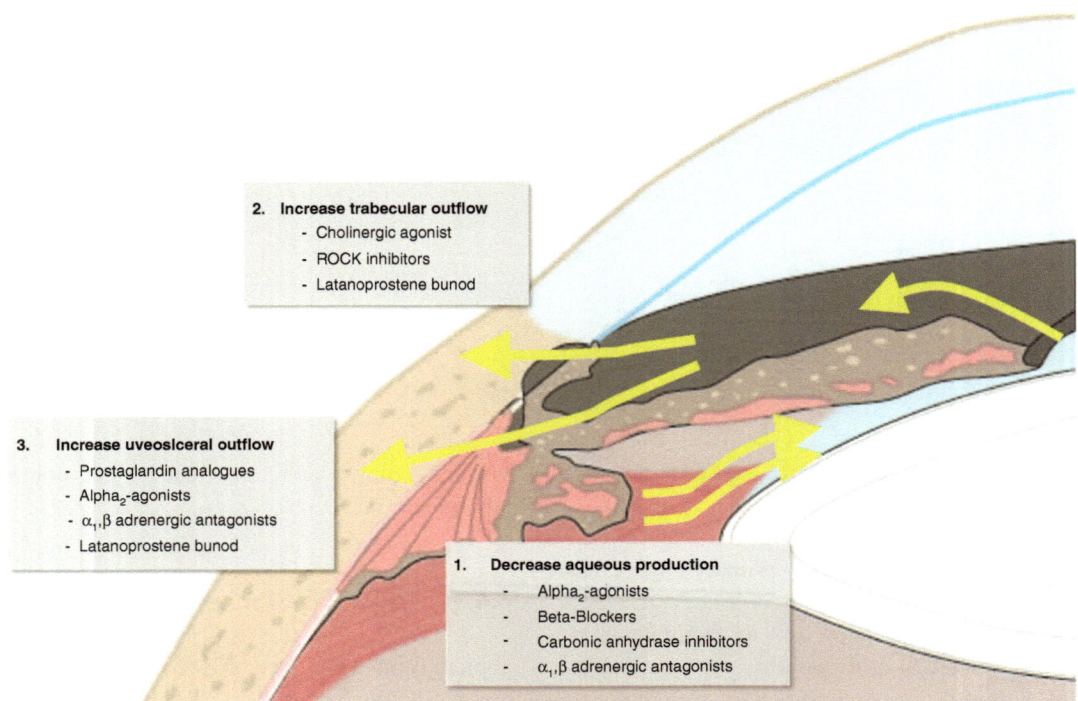

Fig. 4.1 Glaucoma medications/classes and IOP reduction mechanisms

though significantly more stinging or irritating than the control BSS. The data may be beneficial in selecting an agent for those experiencing problems of ocular discomfort from beta-blockers.

In acute settings, timolol is usually used to reduce IOP before a definitive laser or surgical management. The role in chronic angle closure glaucoma is well established as this agent is more effective than pilocarpine, and has an additive effect when combined with other classes of anti-glaucoma drugs. However, tachyphylaxis and long-term drift can decrease the efficacy in a significant number of cases.

Awareness of ß-blockers' local and systemic side effects is important. Ocular side effects are uncommon. Systemic side effects are far more significant. Life-threatening complications such as severe bradycardia, arrhythmias, heart failure, and severe bronchospasm have been associated with topical therapy. These agents should, therefore, be avoided in patients with severe heart disease, asthma, or chronic pulmonary disease [8].

ß-blocker is commonly combined with other classes of hypotensive medication. There are many fixed combination drugs available, namely timolol-dorzolamide, timolol-brinzolamide, timolol-brimonidine, timolol-prostaglandin, and timolol-pilocarpine. The fixed combination drugs achieve greater IOP reduction than any individual agent while reducing the number of drops, reducing the potential toxicity of preservative, avoiding the washout effect, and could improve compliance [9].

4.4.2 Prostaglandins

Prostaglandins reduce IOP by increasing uveoscleral outflow. Clinically, there are 4 prostaglandin analogues (PGA) that are commonly prescribed, namely latanoprost, bimatoprost, travoprost, and tafluprost. It is generally accepted that PGA is the most effective topical ocular hypotensive drugs in primary open angle glaucoma (POAG) and ocular hypertension (OHT) [1]. For primary angle closure (PAC) and primary angle closure glaucoma (PACG), all PGAs have been shown to be effective as well. For example, youngest PGA (tafluprost) in real-world settings also showed that its IOP lowering efficacy in PACG/PAC after iridotomy with at least 90 degrees of visible trabecular meshwork. It was not significantly different from what was shown in POAG/OHT subjects up to 12 months [10]. For CACG, earlier studies demonstrated that PGA, like latanoprost was more effective than ß-blocker, in randomized control studies [11, 12]. In a crossover comparative study, the mean IOP reductions were greater with 0.005% latanoprost (8.2 mmHg) once daily than 0.5% timolol twice daily (6.1 mmHg) when used as primary therapy in CACG after a laser iridotomy [13]. Based on a systematic review, the safety and efficacy of latanoprost as monotherapy for CACG is superior to timolol as latanoprost can reduce mean IOP by more than 30% while timolol is usually in the range of more than 20%. The most frequent ocular adverse effects were ocular hyperemia, discomfort, and blurred vision in a range of less than 10% [14].

For other PGA, there are several studies which also confirm the superior hypotensive efficacy of other PGAs over timolol in CACG. For example, in an early study comparing 0.03% bimatoprost to timolol at 3 months post-treatment, we found 28.3% vs. 18.4% IOP reduction [15]. A longer-term study at 3 years found that bimatoprost 0.03% monotherapy significantly lowers IOP in both POAG and CACG eyes with 50% and 40% chance of having an IOP of <18 mmHg, respectively. However, the upward drift in IOP after 36 months occurred and was higher in the CACG (3.6 mmHg), compared to the POAG (2.1 mmHg), but this was not statistically significant between the groups [16]. Another study that was exclusively looking into patients with 360 degrees synechial closure and no visual potential demonstrated that bimatoprost 0.03% treatment demonstrated a statistically significant IOP reduction [17]. When compared with latanoprost, we found that 0.004% travoprost provided equal or a slightly greater diurnal IOP control (at 4 PM time point) than 0.005% latanoprost at a short-term (12 weeks) study [18]. Another study

reported that both agents significantly reduced IOP in CACG after LPI, and there was no significant difference in IOP reduction between the two treatments [19]. Based on meta-analysis, all PGAs are effective and superior to timolol in CACG. Perhaps travoprost and bimatoprost are slightly superior to latanoprost, but latanoprost is better tolerated [20]. It is not clear that whether the difference in hypotensive efficacy between different PGA is due to pre-treatment IOP (selection bias) or heterogenicity of CACG (different CACG subtype and severity), or the different PGA molecule in the different studies. What seems universal is PGA does lower IOP in CACG and even in acute attack or eye with no visible ciliary-body face with 360 degrees of PAS and IOP greater than 21 mmHg without medication [21]. In practice, we may prescribe any PGA in CACG based on availability, healthcare system, national drug list, temperature-sensitive issue, local side effect, and individual preference.

When compared with drugs in other groups, latanoprost monotherapy is shown to be more effective than unfixed combination therapy with 0.5% timolol maleate and 1% dorzolamide in the treatment of CACG following relief of pupillary block [22].

The mechanism of action of PGA in angle closure is not specifically studied, but it could at least work in the same way as in OAG. It is postulated that PGA enhanced aqueous access to the ciliary body by way of the still-open part of the angle, through the iris, or across the iris root. By analyzing the EXACT study data [12], we can investigate into the relationship between the configuration of the drainage angle and the IOP lowering efficacy of latanoprost in subjects with chronic angle closure glaucoma. It was shown that IOP-lowering efficacy of latanoprost was not affected by the degree of angle narrowing or extent of synechial closure [23]. The delayed onset of action does not preclude its use in AAC but the hypotensive effect could be variable.

Systemic side effects of topical PGAs are minimal, whereas local side effects are relatively common. Conjunctival hyperemia, thicker and longer eyelashes, iris hyperpigmentation, periocular skin darkening are commonly reported [24].

The rate of these occurrences depends on PGA type and its concentration. Active ingredients were deemed responsible for the hyperemia. Deepening of Upper Eyelid Sulcus (DUES), in combination with other clinical findings (mild ptosis, sunken eyeball, or enophthalmos), was later described as Prostaglandin Associated Periorbitopathy (PAP) which is another kind of local effects notorious for PGAs [25]. This periorbital effect is not only of cosmetic concern but also leading to the difficulties in eye examination and surgery due to lid and orbital tightness. It was postulated that PGA molecules penetrate periocular tissue to act on its receptor on adipocyte surface and inhibit lipogenesis [26]. The cells shrunk, causing reduction of periocular tissue volume and the eyeball consequently sunk in. Nevertheless, it is reversible once the suspicious PGA stopped. Some studies showed that switching to another type in its class may be sufficient to change the course [27]. Factors related to PAP were also studied. Age over 60 years, less BMI, 0.03% bimatoprost, 0.04% travoprost, or the use with timolol, but not with gender or duration of use, was reported at a higher chance to develop PAP [28].

4.4.3 Carbonic Anhydrase Inhibitors

Carbonic anhydrase inhibitors (CAIs) are sulfonamide drugs that lower IOP by reducing aqueous humor formation. In the ciliary epithelium, carbonic anhydrase isoenzyme II catalyzes the conversion of CO_2 and H_2O to HCO_3 and H^+, a process important for the production of aqueous humor. By inhibiting this conversion, aqueous production is interrupted. To achieve the therapeutic effect, more than 90% of the CA activity needs to be inhibited. CAIs are available as both systemic (oral or intravenous) and topical agents.

4.4.3.1 Systemic CAIs

Acetazolamide is widely used and is very effective for the treatment of acute angle closure (glaucoma). The traditional oral dosage in adults is 250 mg tablets every 6 hour or 500 mg sustained-release capsules twice each day. Ocular hypotensive effect of tablets peaks in 2 hour and lasts up to 6 hours, whereas that of capsule peaks in 8 hour and persists beyond 12 hours.

Intravenous acetazolamide provides a more rapid onset. A peak effect reaches within 15 min, and the duration lasts for 4 h. For acute angle closure, it is given with a dosage of 250 mg IV. The rapid reduction of aqueous production in the posterior chamber creates the pressure gradient between the anterior and posterior chamber. This results in a concave iris configuration and, in the absence of PAS, the angle widens.

The long-term usage is limited from their numerous adverse effects. Paresthesia, taste disturbance, nausea, vomiting, fatigue, and weight loss are all common. Potential life-threatening complications are rare but should be more cautious in patients with cardiorespiratory, renal disorders, and preexisting electrolytes abnormalities because the drug can induce metabolic acidosis, hypokalemia, and hyponatremia. Other serious complications include severe allergic reaction, Steven-Johnson syndrome, aplastic anemia, thrombocytopenia, and agranulocytosis [29].

A clinician must be aware that acetazolamide has a paradoxical effect by inducing choroidal effusion, a non-pupillary block mechanism, leading to angle closure. The exact mechanism of how choroidal effusion is induced is not clearly understood but shallowing of the anterior chamber, swelling of the lens, myopic shift, and retinal edema had been reported [30]. There are a few case reports of acute bilateral angle closure following cataract surgery [31, 32]. Acetazolamide is also a sulfa-based agent with potential cross reactivity with topiramate and hydrochorothiazide.

4.4.3.2 Topical CAIs

Topical CAIs are better tolerated than systemic form. The IOP-lowering efficacy is comparable to alpha$_2$-agonists. Dorzolamide is available as 2% and brinzolamide as a 1% eye drop. The recommended dosage is three times daily for dorzolamide and twice daily for brinzolamide. These agents often are available as a fixed combination drug with ß-blockers and alpha$_2$-agonists.

Side effects of topical CAIs are ocular discomfort (stinging, burning, and foreign body sensation), dry eyes, and blepharitis. Irreversible corneal decompensation has been reported in patients with marked endothelial compromise [33]. But another study showed no effect on corneal endothelial morphology after receiving 1% dorzolamide for 3 months in glaucoma patients [34]. So it is not an absolute contraindication to prescribe topical CAI, but ophthalmologists should be aware of this potential side effect when there is a coexisting corneal problem, especially in post-penetrating keratoplasty cases. Unfortunately, secondary angle closure is quite common in the post-keratoplasty procedure. In practice, topical CAI is not prescribed as a first-line medication in ACG but usually after PGA and ß-blockers. The fixed combination is commonly prescribed when there is an additional IOP required. If there is a contraindication of ß-blockers, a fixed combination brinzolamide and brimonidine are also available.

4.4.4 Selective Adrenergic Agonists

Selective adrenergic agonists reduce IOP by suppressing aqueous humor production. Apraclonidine and brimonidine are alpha-2 agonists in clinical use. Brimonidine appears to produce an increased uveoscleral outflow in addition to inhibit aqueous production, so-called dual action [35]. There is suggestive evidence that brimonidine is neuroprotective. The advantage of these agents is that they lower IOP rapidly and substantially within 1 hour after instillation. This makes it a potentially useful drug for acute angle closure. Moreover, these agents are also useful in the prophylaxis of post-laser iridotomy and trabeculoplasty IOP spike [36]. Brimonidine 0.2% was found to have an efficacy comparable to that of apraclonidine 1.0% in preventing post-LPI IOP spikes and did not have a pupil dilating effect [37].

One study comparing the effect of brimonidine and timolol in reducing visual field loss in patients with acute primary angle closure, suggested that there was no difference in the prevalence of visual field defects or rate of visual field progression between brimonidine and timolol treated groups [38]. Few clinical data describe using adrenergic agonists in CACG. A report found that brimonidine used as adjunctive treatment to timolol was well tolerated and provided additive IOP reduc-

tion in POAG and CACG at the same level; 19.4% and 20.1%, respectively [39].

Local side effects consist of conjunctival hyperemia, blurring, follicular conjunctivitis, and allergic reaction. Systemic adverse effects include dry mouth, headache, and fatigue. Unlike clonidine, cardiovascular effects are rarely seen with selective alpha$_2$-agonists [40].

At present, there are two commercially available concentrations of brimonidine, 0.15% (with stabilized oxychloro complex preservative) and 0.2% (with benzalkonium chloride preservative), as well as a fixed combination form of timolol-brimonidine and brimonidine-brinzolamide. There is suggestive evidence, as well as clinical experience, that the higher the concentration, the more likely the ocular allergic reaction [41]. The fixed combination seems to be more tolerated, in terms of ocular allergy, than a monotherapy with brimonidine [42].

4.4.5 Miotics (Cholinergic Agents)

Pilocarpine, the most commonly prescribed cholinergic compound, works by contracting the iris sphincter, thus pulling the peripheral iris from trabecular meshwork, opening the angle, and increasing aqueous outflow through the trabecular meshwork. This agent also causes ciliary muscle contraction, which resulting in narrowing of the angle and shallowing of the anterior chamber [43] from the anterior movement of the lens–iris diaphragm. This may paradoxically worsen the pupillary block and further angle closure if there is another mechanism, like lens-induced or ciliary block mechanism involved. Another disadvantage is that it is ineffective in eyes with high IOP because iris sphincter becomes ischemic and paralyzed.

Pilocarpine is recommended in typical cases of acute angle closure when the IOP was reduced by other medications to the level that the iris sphincter can respond to the drug. Constriction of pupil facilitates in performing laser iridotomy. Careful examination to rule out lens-related mechanism as pilocarpine can induce even acute attack if there is an abnormal lens position or morphology [44].

The chronic usage of pilocarpine in CACG is rare because this agent reduces the uveoscleral outflow. For this reason, its action may actually worsen glaucoma if used in patients with little to no trabecular outflow. A study revealed pilocarpine could have no effect on or even increased IOP in chronic angle closure eyes of different pathological mechanisms [45].

Ocular adverse effects are dimmed or blurred vision from miosis and induced accommodative myopia, brow ache, and rarely retinal detachment. Systemic side effects are not common but can include salivation, sweating, diarrhea, abdominal cramps, and bradycardia [46].

In practice, pilocarpine may be helpful in eyes with plateau iris syndrome but should not be given as a routine to all CACG eyes. Avoid pilocarpine if there is a lens mechanism or ciliary block mechanism identified as it will further narrowing the angle. The benefit of IOP lowering in angle closure is usually seen in aphakic or pseudophakic eye after the lens has been removed and the angle is widen. So the trabecular outflow can be enhanced with less angle blockage.

4.4.6 Hyperosmotic Agents

Hyperosmotic agents, given systemically, raise blood osmolality and create an osmotic gradient that draws water from the vitreous cavity. The reduction of vitreous volume allows the lens to move posteriorly, which deepens the anterior chamber and opens the angle. So there is a strong implication for acute angle closure. With time, a variable amount of the hyperosmotic agent may enter the eye. This equilibrium between the two compartments reduces the efficacy of the drug. Patients should be instructed to limit ingestion of fluid after administration of these agents because fluid intake decreases the drug-induced hyperosmolality [47].

Oral hyperosmotic agents include glycerol (50% solution), which is usually administered at 1–1.5 g/kg, and isosorbide, at 1.5–2 g/kg. The ocular hypotensive effect of glycerol peaks in 30 min and lasts for 5 hours. However, glycerol can induce hyperglycemia, particularly in diabetic patients. To reduce this unfavorable effect, it may be more suitable to employ isosorbide which is not metabolized to glucose in this regard. In angle closure glaucoma, hyperosmotic agents are of greatest value in an acute attack. Many ophthalmologists keep oral glycerol in their offices for use in such cases. The other indication of glycerin solution is to clear the cornea before LPI. The cornea can be edematous and hazy in AAC. By instilling a drop of glycerin on the cornea after topical anesthesia, can immediately clear the cornea to allow LPI or laser iridoplasty. The hyperosmotic nature of glycerin can cause significant irritation and discomfort but very effective in temporary clear the cornea for an urgent laser treatment or even paracentesis.

Intravenous mannitol is considered in acute glaucoma presenting with vomiting. A dosage of 1–2 g/kg of body weight of a 20% solution given in 30–45 min has been suggested. The maximal effect occurs within 1 hour, and the duration varies from 2 to 6 hours [48].

Side effects with hyperosmotic agents are common and can be serious or even fatal. Headaches, nausea, and vomit are the most frequent. Electrolyte imbalance, leading to hyponatremia or hyperkalemia, is often associated with mannitol. This is transient and usually of no consequence. The devastating complications, such as pulmonary edema is mostly associated with large dose administration. Congestive heart failure subsequent to hyperkalemia or acute renal failure may be precipitated in patients with borderline cardiac and renal status [49].

4.4.7 Intravenous Lidocaine

Lidocaine is a widely used anesthetic agent frequently employed to attenuate the increase in intracranial pressure and IOP of patients receiving succinylcholine prior to intubation. For this reason, there was a study investigating the effectiveness of a combination of both intravenous injection of lidocaine and IOP-lowering medications, in refractory AAC. Each patient received topical pilocarpine, timolol, systemic acetazolamide, and mannitol as primary treatment but

IOP was still high after 4 h with mean 50 mmHg. After the administration of intravenous lidocaine, the mean IOP was reduced to 39 mmHg at 30 min and 24 mmHg at 2 hour with instant symptomatic relief for all patients [50]. In spite of this, the exact efficacy and safety need further investigation in large case studies. At the moment, this is not a standard practice in ACG.

4.4.8 Steroid

Anterior chamber inflammation is often related to AAC. The scale is usually proportional to the severity and duration of the course. Inflammation can also promote the development of PAS, which results in chronic elevation of IOP. Intensive topical steroid is recommended in addition to antiglaucoma. Besides, it is used for the short-term to prevent IOP elevation after anterior segment laser procedures.

4.5 Novel Antiglaucoma Medications

4.5.1 ROCK Inhibitors

Ripasudil is a Rho-kinase (ROCK) inhibitor approved in 2014 to be used clinically as an ocular hypotensive agent. Study in animal models showed that it increased trabecular meshwork outflow facility by decreasing actin stress fibers and myosin light-chain phosphorylation as well as increased Schlemm's canal endothelial cell permeability. Widening of the extracellular spaces at the optically empty area of the juxtacanalicular tissue was also observed. The process led to increasing conventional outflow, followed by decreasing intraocular pressure [51].

Ripasudil showed its IOP-lowering effects when applied as a single drug or in combination with beta-blockers or PGA analogs. The recommended dosage is twice daily. Conjunctival hyperemia, conjunctivitis, and blepharitis were the most common adverse drug reactions (ADRs) [52].

Netarsudil is another ROCK inhibitor approved in 2017 with once-daily dosing, mainly used in the USA, whereas Ripasudil is more favorable in Japan. Combined fixed-dose Netarsudil and Latanoprost were shown in a short-term study that it had relatively superior IOP reduction efficacy compared to its individual active agents at the same concentration. Conjunctival hyperemia was not significantly increased when two drugs combined [53].

ROCK inhibitors were primarily investigated in POAG or OHT. Interestingly, a post-marketing surveillance study in Japan recruited 54 PACG eyes out of the eligible 2839 eyes for the analysis. Ripasudil was shown to be able to significantly reduce IOP in angle closure (from $22.2 + 8.5$ mmHg baseline to $16.6 + 4.5$ mmHg at 3 months). The adverse drug reactions were noted 8% locally, most of them apparently were conjunctival hyperemia and conjunctivitis. Non-ocular side effects were found less than 0.1% [54].

4.5.2 Nitric Oxide Donating Agents

Latanoprostene bunod (LBN), a nitric oxide (NO) donating PGA, reduces IOP by increase the uveoscleral outflow pathway and also enhance the conventional outflow. In essence, LBN has dual mechanism, dual pathway because of the linked molecule. Latanoprost is known to upregulate matrix metalloproteinase expression leading to remodeling of extracellular matrix at ciliary muscle, thus increase the uveoscleral outflow. While the linked NO-donating moiety to latanoprost, induce cytoskeletal relaxation via the soluble guanylyl cyclase-cyclic guanosine monophosphate (sGC-cGMP) signaling pathway. The NO help relaxing trabecular meshwork and Schlemm's channel, improves the conventional pathway [55].

The enzyme NO synthase is mainly discovered in the anterior segment, nonpigmented epithelium of ciliary processes, ciliary muscles, trabecular meshwork, Schlemm's canal, and collector channels, all of which respond to synthesized NO efficiently. NO can relax trabecular meshwork, facilitating aqueous outflow. Since NO can relieve vascular muscle tone, it was postulated that NO could regulate ocular vascular blood flow and may, in turn, protect retinal ganglion cells. Markers for NO were found decreasing in glaucoma subjects.

Overall adverse effects of LBN 0.024% solution applied topically once daily are similar to those with latanoprost. Conjunctival hyperemia is the most commonly reported adverse reaction [56].

Nipradilol is an alpha/beta-adrenergic blocker with NO donating releasing action. It reduces aqueous production by the action through the β-blocking property and aggravates aqueous drainage through uveoscleral passage [57]. Dosage is 0.25%, twice daily. The hypotensive effect was reported in normal-tension glaucoma, improved ocular vasodilation via the action of donated nitric oxide (NO) was also shown [58].

Studies of both agents are limited to POAG or OHT. Up until now, there is no study of their efficacy in ACG. By the assumption that if the mechanical blockage is corrected, partially or completely, the dual action may provide an additional hypotensive effect. But this remains unproven until properly studied.

4.5.3 Cannabinoids

There are two active compounds of cannabinoids, tetrahydrocannabinol (THC) and cannabidiol (CBD), found to have medical advantages. THC is responsible for psychotropic effects, appetite stimulation, and control of nausea and vomiting. CBD may mitigate musculo-spasm and chronic pain. Cannabinoids ocular hypotensive effects, mainly by THC, was believed to have resulted from its action through endocannabinoid receptors (CB1, GPR18) in the structures such as trabecular meshwork, Sclemm's canal, and ciliary body [59]. Inhaled, oral, or intravenous administration could carry this effect. Ocular hypotension was temporarily achieved, maximum at 60–90 min, and lasted for only 4–5 h compared to

vehicles [60]. Despite those findings, the IOP lowering mechanism of cannabinoids has not yet been determined. The topical route was not able to show a satisfactory outcome as cannabinoids are lipophilic, resulting in difficulty in corneal penetration and likely to have an inverse effect on the corneal surface. On the other hand, CBD was revealed to have an opposing effect as CB1 antagonist, elevating IOP in rats after 4 h post-administration and hampering THC IOP lowering activity.

Amount consumed to reach a brief ocular hypotensive effect can lead to undesirable neuro-psychological and behavioral effects. This precludes cannabinoids from being licensed to clinical practice by several leading national ophthalmology societies [61, 62]. There is no reported study on cannabinoids use in ACG.

Since Cannabinoids have not been approved for glaucoma treatment, its activity is not tabulated.

4.6 Medical Management in the Different Clinical Setting

4.6.1 Acute Angle Closure

In Acute Angle Closure (AAC), IOP rises rapidly, and the patients usually suffer from severe symptoms. The main purpose of medical therapy is to reduce IOP as quickly as possible, relieve ocular pain and headache, and control ocular inflammation. When the cornea clears enough after IOP reduction, laser iridotomy can be performed, and the attack can be broken. The faster the IOP reduction, the lesser the damage to the optic nerve and iris.

Systemic medications have a very rapid onset and powerful IOP reduction. Oral glycerol and acetazolamide are the agents usually used. If the patients vomited, the intravenous route (mannitol or IV acetazolamide) should be considered.

In practice, the following regimen can be considered:

- Topical ß-blockers, i.e., timolol start immediately, then every 12 h.
- Topical alpha$_2$-agonist like brimonidine immediately, then every 8 h.
- Oral Diamox (check if any sulfa hypersensitivity) 1–2 tablets depending on the body weight, then every 6 h.
- Oral glycerin mixed with lemon juice or other juice if IOP is extremely high and with corneal edema. If the patient has nausea and vomiting, one may consider intravenous mannitol and anti-emetics.
- Topical pilocarpine must be used selectively and as a second-line drug after the cornea becomes clear enough and to prepare the eye for LPI or laser iridoplasty.
- Analgesic drug and topical steroid.

Re-evaluate the patient in 45 minutes. If there is no response, other surgical interventions like paracentesis or immediate laser iridoplasty or LPI should be considered.

4.6.2 Chronic Angle Closure Glaucoma

The principles of medical treatment for CACG are similar to POAG. Nevertheless, LPI, laser iridoplasty, or lens surgery must be performed to remove the mechanical blockage in conjunction with medical treatment. Besides reducing the IOP, LPI also protects an acute attack of angle closure and prevents the development of synechiae closure.

Most available medications are proved to be effective in CACG, including PGAs. It is quite common that CACG patients will need more than monotherapy. If the patient is taking PGA, there is a potential detrimental effect of pilocarpine on the PGA. Also, if patients have extensive PAS, treatment by pilocarpine may worsen the condition.

Other aspects of chronic medical treatment are long-term side effects of medications, compliance of the patients, systemic health, and affordability.

4.6.3 Prophylaxis for IOP Spikes After Laser

IOP spikes can occur after anterior segment laser on iris or drainage angle. The preoperative outflow facility is directly related to the maximum postoperative IOP elevation. Causes of IOP spikes may be from pigment dispersion, protein, and inflammatory cells that further impede aqueous outflow.

Alpha$_2$-agonists, apraclonidine, and brimonidine are commonly used and effective in preventing IOP spikes. Many studies reported that the efficacy between both drugs is not different [63]. These agents can be administered before or immediately after performing laser.

Pretreatment with latanoprost in Nd:YAG LPI was associated with an increase mean IOP 2.5 mmHg at 1 hour and 0.8 mmHg at 2 hour, but less than pretreatment with pilocarpine. 23% of the latanoprost group developed a rise in IOP more than 6 mmHg, whereas 42% in pilocarpine did. Although latanoprost may reduce the pressure rise following LPI, its application is limited by a late onset of effect [64].

4.6.4 Plateau Iris

Peripheral laser iridoplasty outcome seems variable. The direct-acting cholinergic agent like pilocarpine has been described to be effective in increasing the angle opening.

4.7 Summary

Medical treatment plays an important role in the management of ACG, both in AAC and in CACG. In AAC, medical treatment prepares the eye for laser treatment (LPI and iridoplasty) and reduces IOP to preserve ocular microstructures and the optic nerve. But even after successful LPI or lens surgery, a significant number of CACG patients will have persistent IOP elevation, which must be treated with medications. Most available hypotensive agents are effective in CACG except for the new drugs that either little or no efficacy data available in ACG. Many CACG will need multiple medications. There are plenty of fixed combination drugs that help to reduce the need for multiple drops and could minimize adverse events while enhancing compliance. The role of medications in ACG can be slightly different in certain clinical settings of ACG. Efficacy and adverse effects of each agent should be considered individually when choosing the treatment, especially when a long-term continuation is needed.

Acknowledgment Patcharaporn Jaru-ampornpan, MD. for contribution on table and figure.

References

1. Asia Pacific Glaucoma Society. Asia pacific glaucoma guidelines. Amsterdam: Kugler Publications; 2016.
2. Rutkowski PC, Thompson HS. Mydriasis and increased intraocular pressure. Arch Ophthalmol. 1972;87:21–4.
3. Sng CC, Aquino MC, Liao J, Zheng C, Ang M, Chew PT. Anterior segment morphology after acute primary angle closure treatment: a randomised study comparing iridoplasty and medical therapy. Br J Ophthalmol. 2016;100(4):542–8.
4. Lai JS, Tham CC, Chua JK, et al. To compare argon laser peripheral iridoplasty (ALPI) against systemic medications in treatment of acute primary angle-closure: mid-term results. Eye. 2006;20(3):309–14.
5. Cai W, Lou Q, Fan J, Yu D, Shen T, Yu J. Efficacy and safety of argon laser peripheral Iridoplasty and systemic medical therapy in Asian patients with acute primary angle closure: a meta-analysis of randomized controlled trials. J Ophthalmol. 2019;2019:7697416.
6. Kumar RS, Tantisevi V, Wong MH, et al. Plateau Iris in Asian subjects with primary angle closure Glaucoma. Arch Ophthalmol. 2009;127(10):1269–72.
7. Liu JH, Kripke DF, Weinreb RN. Comparison of the nocturnal effects of once-daily timolol and latanoprost on intraocular pressure. Am J Ophthalmol. 2004;138(3):389–95.
8. Mirza GE, Karaküçük S, Temel E. Comparison of the effects of 0.5% timolol maleate, 2% carteolol hydrochloride, and 0.3% metipranolol on intraocular pressure and perimetry findings and evaluation of their ocular and systemic effects. J Glaucoma. 2000;9(1):45–50.
9. Holló G, Topouzis F, Fechtner RD. Fixed-combination intraocular pressure-lowering therapy for glaucoma and ocular hypertension: advantages in clinical practice. Expert Opin Pharmacother. 2014;15(12):1737–47.
10. Tumbocon JA, Macasaet AM. Efficacy and safety of tafluprost 0.0015% - retrospective analysis of real-world data from the Philippines. Clin Ophthalmol. 2019;13:1627–34.
11. Aung T, Wong HT, Yip CC, Leong JY, Chan YH, Chew PT. Comparison of the intraocular pressure-lowering effect of latanoprost and timolol in patients with chronic angle closure glaucoma: a preliminary study. Ophthalmology. 2000;107(6):1178–83.
12. Chew PT, Aung T, Aquino MV, Rojanapongpun P, Group ES. Intraocular pressure-reducing effects and safety of latanoprost versus timolol in patients with chronic angle-closure glaucoma. Ophthalmology. 2004;111(3):427–34.
13. Sihota R, Saxena R, Agarwal HC, et al. Crossover comparison of timolol and latanoprost in chronic primary angle-closure glaucoma. Arch Ophthalmol. 2004;122(2):185–9.
14. Chen R, Yang K, Zheng Z, Ong ML, Wang NL, Zhan SY. Meta-analysis of the efficacy and safety of Latanoprost Monotherapy in patients with angle-closure Glaucoma. J Glaucoma. 2016;25(3):e134–44.
15. RojanaPongpun P, Pandav SS, Reyes MR, Euswas A. Comparison of the efficacy and safety of bimatoprost and timolol for treatment of chronic angle closure glaucoma. Asian J Ophthalmol. 2007;9(6):239–44.
16. Gupta V, Srinivasan G, Sharma A, et al. Comparative evaluation of bimatoprost monotherapy in primary chronic angle closure and primary open angle glaucoma eyes: a three-year study. J Ocul Pharmacol Ther. 2007;23(4):351–8.
17. Vyas P, Naik U, Gangaiah JB. Efficacy of bimatoprost 0.03% in reducing intraocular pressure in patients with 360 degrees synechial angle-closure glaucoma: a preliminary study. Indian J Ophthalmol. 2011;59(1):13–6.
18. Chew PTK, RojanaPongpun P, Euswas A, Lu D, Chua J, Hui S, et al. Intraocular pressure-lowering effect and safety of travoprost 0.004% and latanoprost 0.005% for the treatment of chronic angle closure glaucoma. Asian J Ophthalmol. 2006;8(1):13–9.
19. Chen MJ, Chen YC, Chou CK, Hsu WM. Comparison of the effects of latanoprost and travoprost on intraocular pressure in chronic angle-closure glaucoma. J Ocul Pharmacol Ther. 2006;22(6):449–54.
20. Li J, Lin X, Yu M. Meta-analysis of randomized controlled trials comparing latanoprost with other glaucoma medications in chronic angle-closure glaucoma. Eur J Ophthalmol. 2015;25(1):18–26.
21. Kook MS, Cho HS, Yang SJ, Kim S, Chung J. Efficacy of latanoprost in patients with chronic angle-closure glaucoma and no visible ciliary-body face: a preliminary study. J Ocul Pharmacol Ther. 2005;21(1):75–84.
22. Sakai H, Shinjyo S, Nakamura Y, Nakamura Y, Ishikawa S, Sawaguchi S. Comparison of latanoprost monotherapy and combined therapy of 0.5% timolol and 1% dorzolamide in chronic primary angle-closure

glaucoma (CACG) in Japanese patients. J Ocul Pharmacol Ther. 2005;21(6):483–9.

23. Aung T, Chan YH, Chew PT, Group ES. Degree of angle closure and the intraocular pressure-lowering effect of latanoprost in subjects with chronic angle-closure glaucoma. Ophthalmology. 2005;112(2):267–71.

24. Alm A, Grierson I, Shields MB. Side effects associated with prostaglandin analog therapy. Surv Ophthalmol. 2008;53(Suppl 1):S93–S105.

25. Kucukevcilioglu M, Bayer A, Uysal Y, et al. Prostaglandin associated periorbitopathy in patients using bimatoprost, latanoprost and travoprost. Clin Exp Ophthalmol. 2014;42:126–31.

26. Taketani Y, Yamagishi R, Fujishiro T, et al. Activation of the prostanoid FP receptor inhibits adipogenesis leading to deepening of the upper eyelid sulcus in prostaglandin-associated periorbitopathy. Invest Ophthalmol Vis Sci. 2014;55:1269–76.

27. Sakata R, Shirato S, Miyata K, et al. Recovery from deepening of the upper eyelid sulcus after switching from bimatoprost to latanoprost. Jpn J Ophthalmol. 2013;57:179–84.

28. Patradul C, Tantisevi V, Manassakorn A. Factors related to prostaglandin-associated Periorbitopathy in Glaucoma patients. Asia Pac J Ophthalmol (Phila). 2017;6(3):238–42.

29. Van Berkel MA, Elefritz JL. Evaluating off-label uses of acetazolamide. Am J Health Syst Pharm. 2018;75(8):524–31.

30. Lee GC, Tam CP, Danesh-Meyer HV, Myers JS, Katz LJ. Bilateral angle closure glaucoma induced by sulphonamide-derived medications. Clin Exp Ophthalmol. 2007;35:55–8.

31. Parthasarathi S, Myint K, Singh G, Mon S, Sadasivam P, Dhillon B. Bilateral acetazolamide-induced choroidal effusion following cataract surgery. Eye (Lond). 2007 Jun;21(6):870–2.

32. Mancino R, Varesi C, Cerulli A, Aiello F, Nucci C. Acute bilateral angle-closure glaucoma and choroidal effusion associated with acetazolamide administration after cataract surgery. J Cataract Refract Surg. 2011 Feb;37(2):415–7.

33. Konowal A, Morrison JC, Brown SV, et al. Irreversible corneal decompensation in patients treated with topical dorzolamide. Am J Ophthalmol. 1999;127(4):403–6.

34. Inoue K, Okugawa K, Oshika T, et al. Influence of dorzolamide on corneal endothelium. Jpn J Ophthalmol. 2003;47(2):129–33.

35. Toris CB, Gleason ML, Camras CB, Yablonski ME. Effects of brimonidine on aqueous humor dynamics in human eyes. Arch Ophthalmol. 1995;113(12):1514–7.

36. Zhang L, Weizer JS, Musch DC. Perioperative medications for preventing temporarily increased intraocular pressure after laser trabeculoplasty. Cochrane Database Syst Rev 2017;2(2):CD010746. Published 2017 Feb 23.

37. Yuen NS, Cheung P, Hui SP. Comparing brimonidine 0.2% to apraclonidine 1.0% in the prevention of intraocular pressure elevation and their pupillary effects following laser peripheral iridotomy. Jpn J Ophthalmol. 2005;49(2):89–92.

38. Aung T, Oen FT, Wong HT, et al. Randomised controlled trial comparing the effect of brimonidine and timolol on visual field loss after acute primary angle closure. Br J Ophthalmol. 2004;88(1):88–94.

39. Ruangvaravate N, Kitnarong N, Metheetrairut A, et al. Efficacy of brimonidine 0.2 per cent as adjunctive therapy to beta-blockers: a comparative study between POAG and CACG in Asian eyes. J Med Assoc Thail. 2002;85(8):894–900.

40. Cantor LB. The evolving pharmacotherapeutic profile of brimonidine, an alpha 2-adrenergic agonist, after four years of continuous use. Expert Opin Pharmacother. 2000;1(4):815–34.

41. Sullivan-Mee M, Pensyl D, Alldredge B, Halverson K, Gerhardt G, Qualls C. Brimonidine hypersensitivity when switching between 0.2% and 0.15% formulations. J Ocul Pharmacol Ther. 2010;26(4):355–60.

42. Motolko MA. Comparison of allergy rates in glaucoma patients receiving brimonidine 0.2% monotherapy versus fixed-combination brimonidine 0.2%-timolol 0.5% therapy. Curr Med Res Opin. 2008;24(9):2663–7.

43. Hung L, Yang CH, Chen MS. Effect of pilocarpine on anterior chamber angles. J Ocul Pharmacol Ther. 1995;11(3):221–6.

44. Day AC, Nolan W, Malik AN, Viswanathan AC, Foster PJ. Pilocarpine induced acute angle closure. BMJ Case Rep. 2012;2012:bcr0120125694corr1.

45. Li M, Yan XQ, Li GY, Zhang H. Post-miosis changes in the anterior chamber structures in primary and lens-induced secondary chronic angle-closure glaucoma. Int J Ophthalmol. 2019;12(4):675–80.

46. Schuman JS. Short- and long-term safety of glaucoma drugs. Expert Opin Drug Saf. 2002;1(2):181–94.

47. Hill K, Whitney J, Trotter R. Intravenous hypertonic urea in the management of angle closure glaucoma. Arch Ophthalmol. 1961;72:491.

48. Hoh S-T, Aung T, Chew PTK. Medical management of angle closure glaucoma. Semin Ophthalmol. 2002;17(2):79–83.

49. Zhang W, Neal J, Lin L, et al. Mannitol in critical care and surgery over 50+ years: a systematic review of randomized controlled trials and complications with meta-analysis. J Neurosurg Anesthesiol. 2019;31(3):273–84.

50. Jin X, Xue A, Zhao Y, et al. Efficacy and safety of intravenous injection of lidocaine in the treatment of acute primary angle-closure glaucoma: a pilot study. Graefes Arch Clin Exp Ophthalmol. 2007;245(11):1611–6.

51. Rao PV, Deng PF, Kumar J, Epstein DL. Modulation of aqueous humor outflow facility by the rho kinase-specific inhibitor Y-27632 [published correction appears in invest Ophthalmol Vis Sci 2001 Jul;42(8):1690]. Invest Ophthalmol Vis Sci. 2001;42(5):1029–37.

52. Tanihara H, Inoue T, Yamamoto T, Kuwayama Y, Abe H, Araie M. Phase 2 randomized clinical study of a rho kinase inhibitor, K-115, in primary open-angle glaucoma and ocular hypertension. Am J Ophthalmol. 2013;156(4):731–6.

53. Lewis RA, Levy B, Ramirez N, et al. Fixed-dose combination of AR-13324 and latanoprost: a double-masked, 28-day, randomised, controlled study in patients with open-angle glaucoma or ocular hypertension [published correction appears in Br J Ophthalmol. 2016 Jul;100(7):1016]. Br J Ophthalmol. 2016;100(3):339–44.

54. Tanihara H, Kakuda T, Sano T, et al. Correction to: safety and efficacy of Ripasudil in Japanese patients with Glaucoma or ocular hypertension: 3-month interim analysis of ROCK-J, a post-marketing surveillance study. Adv Ther. 2019;36(5):1233–4.

55. Kaufman PL. Latanoprostene bunod ophthalmic solution 0.024% for IOP lowering in glaucoma and ocular hypertension. Expert Opin Pharmacother. 2017;18(4):433–44.

56. Mehran NA, Sinha S, Razeghinejad R. New glaucoma medications: latanoprostene bunod, netarsudil, and fixed combination netarsudil-latanoprost. Eye (Lond). 2020 Jan;34(1):72–88.

57. Kanno M, Araie M, Koibuchi H, Masuda K. Effects of topical nipradilol, a beta blocking agent with alpha blocking and nitroglycerin-like activities, on intraocular pressure and aqueous dynamics in humans. Br J Ophthalmol. 2000;84(3):293–9.

58. Inoue K, Noguchi K, Wakakura M, Tomita G. Effect of five years of treatment with nipradilol eye drops in patients with normal tension glaucoma. Clin Ophthalmol. 2011;5:1211–6.

59. Miller S, Daily L, Leishman E, Bradshaw H, Straiker A. Δ9-Tetrahydrocannabinol and Cannabidiol differentially regulate intraocular pressure. Invest Ophthalmol Vis Sci. 2018 Dec 3;59(15):5904–11.

60. Hepler RS, Frank IR. Marihuana smoking and intraocular pressure. JAMA. 1971;217(10):1392.

61. Rafuse P, Buys YM. Medical use of cannabis for glaucoma. Can J Ophthalmol. 2019 Feb;54(1):7–8.

62. American Academy of Ophthalmology. Marijuana in the treatment of glaucoma CTA-2014. Available from: https://www.aao.org/complimentary-therapy-assessment/marijuana-in-treatment-of-glaucoma-cta%2D%2Dmay-2003. Accessed 29 Mar 2020.

63. Chen TC. Brimonidine 0.15% versus apraclonidine 0.5% for prevention of intraocular pressure elevation after anterior segment laser surgery. J Cataract Refract Surg. 2005;31(9):1707–12.

64. Liu CJ, Cheng CY, Chiang SC, et al. Use of latanoprost to reduce acute intraocular pressure rise following neodymium: Yag laser iridotomy. Acta Ophthalmol Scand. 2002;80(3):282–6.

Laser Peripheral Iridotomy

Young Kook Kim and Ki Ho Park

Abstract

Laser peripheral iridotomy (LPI) is a procedure for managing angle-closure glaucoma caused by relative or absolute pupillary block. LPI eliminates pupillary block by allowing the aqueous to pass directly from the posterior chamber into the anterior chamber, bypassing the pupillary opening. LPI allows the iris to flatten, widening the anterior chamber angle, and thus lowering intraocular pressure. It is not common to have complications after LPI; nevertheless, complications are possible following the LPI and careful monitoring is a routine part of the post-procedure care.

Keywords

Laser · Iridotomy · Nd:YAG laser · Argon laser · Indication · Complication · Angle-closure disease

5.1 Introduction

Laser peripheral iridotomy (LPI) is integral to angle-closure disease management. Even though high-energy iridotomy was achieved as early as 1956, its wide application was prevented by frequent iridotomy closure as well as corneal and lenticular damage. From the 1980s, however, Argon and Nd:YAG lasers have allowed LPI to become a routine clinical procedure.

Researches for the fundamental questions related with LPI, such as who can benefit from prophylactic iridotomy, why it fails in some eyes, and what its long-term risks are, especially with regard to cataract formation, have been actively conducted. In this chapter, we review LPI's technical aspects, its uses' indications, as well as potential complications.

Y. K. Kim · K. H. Park (✉)
Department of Medicine, Seoul National University College of Medicine, Seoul, Republic of Korea

Department of Ophthalmology, Seoul National University Hospital, Seoul, Republic of Korea
e-mail: kihopark@snu.ac.kr

© Springer Nature Singapore Pte Ltd. 2021
C. C. Y. Tham (ed.), *Primary Angle Closure Glaucoma (PACG)*,
https://doi.org/10.1007/978-981-15-8120-5_5

5.2   Indications for Laser Peripheral Iridotomy

5.2.1   Acute Angle Closure

The most clear-cut LPI indication is AAC. In AAC eyes, IOP typically is quite high [1, 2], resulting in corneal edema and a mid-dilated pupil. Prior to LPI in AAC eyes, IOP must be lowered sufficiently to ensure a clear cornea. Pre-LPI reduction of IOP has been achieved in 90% of patients using a combination of oral and IV acetazolamide along with topical steroids, pilocarpine, and timolol [3].

In cases of AAC, IOP lowering with LPI frequently is immediate and dramatic. Aung et al. showed that all 110 eyes of Asian patients showed an IOP drop to below 21 mm Hg after patent LPI [2].

Serial gonioscopic examination of AAC eyes after LPI has demonstrated angle widening within the first month. Lim et al. reported angle widening in the first 2 weeks but noted no change for over 1 year afterward [4].

5.2.2   Chronic Angle-Closure Glaucoma

Several studies on patients representative of a variety of ethnic backgrounds have noted IOP lowering after LPI in primary angle-closure glaucoma (PACG) eyes [1, 5–11]. A total of 187 Saudi Arabian PACG eyes showed a significant mean-IOP drop from 24.8 to 17.5 mmHg, equal numbers of patients having received medical therapy 12 months after LPI [1]. A mostly Caucasian population that had been treated with argon LPI for PACG and followed for 53 months showed a mean IOP decrease from 28 to 18.5 mmHg and a medication-number decrease from 1.5 to 0.9 [10]. Another study on 58 Taiwanese PACG eyes reported a mean IOP decrease from 25.4 to 14.1 mmHg over the course of a mean 51-month follow-up period [5].

5.2.3   Primary Angle Closure and Primary Angle-Closure Suspect

The role of LPI in the PAC or PACS treatment algorithm is still debated. When assessing the PAC/PACS for LPI literature, study-subject heterogeneity spanning the entire PAC/PACS spectrum should be considered.

Both short- and long-term changes of anterior-chamber angle width before and after LPI have been evaluated in PAC or PACS eyes (Table 5.1). Short-term angle-width changes in PAC/PACS eyes as evaluated by either gonioscopy or anterior-segment OCT (ASOCT) all showed increased angle width after LPI (Fig. 5.1). In two prospective studies on PACS eyes, long-term angle-width changes were studied for post-LPI follow-up durations up to 18 months [12, 13]. Both studies reported a significant angle-width decrease between post-LPI 2 weeks and 18 months. The Zhongshan Angle Closure Prevention study, meanwhile, included 775 Chinese PACS subjects, each one having been treated by LPI in 1 randomly selected eye, the fellow eye serving as the control [12]. It noted that the LPI-treated eyes showed a much slower rate of angle narrowing over the course of 18 months of follow-up.

5.2.4   Other Indications for Laser Peripheral Iridotomy

Secondary pupillary block resulting from a variety of causes can be relieved by LPI. In aphakic eyes with pupillary block, the vitreous humor forms circumferential adhesions relative to the iris margin. Successful LPI can restore the anterior chamber and lower IOP in cases of aphakia pupillary block, specifically by redirecting the aqueous humor [14].

Pseudophakic pupillary block has been associated with anterior-chamber intraocular lenses (ACIOLs), posterior-chamber intraocular lenses (PCIOLs), and iris fixation lenses [15–17]. Surgical

Table 5.1 Changes in the anterior chamber angle after laser peripheral iridotomy in PAC or PACS

Study (year)	Race	Number of eyes	Angle	Duration	Method of assessment	Angle parameter	Before LPI	After LPI
He (2007)	Chinese	72	ITC ≥ 270	2 weeks	Gonioscopy	Mean Shaffer grade Superior Q	0.4	1.9
						Inferior Q	0.9	2.8
He (2007)	Chinese	72	ITC ≥ 270	2 weeks	UBM	AOD500 (mm)	0.067	0.111
						ARA750 (mm²)	0.04	0.07
Dada (2007)	Indian	54	ITC ≥ 180 PAS(+)	2 weeks	UBM	ITC in ≥ 3 Q	48.60%	18.10%
						AOD500 (mm)	0.107	0.208
						ARA (mm²)	0.132	0.158
Ramani (2009)	Indian	52	ITC ≥ 180	24 months	Gonioscopy	Mean modified Shaffer grade (sup&inf Q)	1	3
How (2012)	96% Chinese	175	ITC ≥ 180	1 week	Gonioscopy	Mean modified Shaffer grade	0.68	1.76
					ASOCT	AOD500 (mm)	0.12	0.19
						ARA (mm²)	0.13	0.17
Lee (2013)	Korean	32	ITC ≥ 270	18 months	ASOCT	AOD750 (mm)	0.17	0.28
						ARA750 (mm²)	0.08	0.13
						Iris curvature (mm)	0.34	0.15
Lin (2013)	Chinese	66	ITC ≥ 270 47% PAS(+)	2 weeks	Gonioscopy	PAS (clock hours)	3	2
					UBM	AOD500 PAS negative (mm)	55.5	75.1
						PAS positive (mm)	38.1	42.0
Jiang (2014)	Chinese	775	ITC ≥ 180	2 weeks	Gonioscopy	Angle width in degrees	13.5	25.7
				18 months	ASOCT	Change in AOD500 (µm)		+54.7
						Change in ARA (×1000 µm²)		+45.2

PAC primary angle closure, *PACS* primary angle-closure suspect, *LPI* laser peripheral iridotomy, *ITC* iridotrabecular contact, *Q* quadrant, *UBM* ultrasound biomicroscopy, *AOD* angle opening distance, *ARA* angle recess area, *PAS* peripheral anterior synechiae

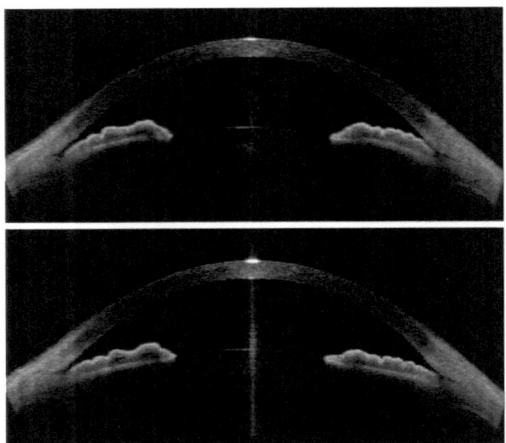

Fig. 5.1 Anterior segment optical coherence tomography images showing anterior chamber configuration before (upper) and after (lower) laser peripheral iridotomy in primary angle-closure suspect

iridectomy during surgery or prophylactic LPI should be considered in order to prevent pupillary block in ACIOLs. Pseudophakic pupillary block arises when aqueous flow from the posterior chamber and the iridocorneal angle are blocked by strong apposition of the pupillary margin to adjacent structures. Several mechanisms, including traumatic intraocular lens (IOL) dislocation, optic capture with in-the-bag haptics, and iris-anterior capsular adhesions, have been reported for cases of pupillary block following PCIOLs [18–20]. Definitive treatment might require IOL replacement and/or repositioning. However, short-term pressure lowering can be achieved, either by mydriasis to dilate the pupil beyond the IOL edges or by LPI for aqueous redirection into the anterior chamber [21, 22]. As for pseudophakic pupillary block, post-LPI recurrence has been reported [23]. Larger size or multiple iridotomies might increase the chance of maintaining route for aqueous flow into the anterior chamber.

Inflammation associated with uveitis potentially causes pupillary block, principally by producing 360 degrees of posterior synechiae and iris bombe. Spencer et al. reviewed 15 eyes of 11 subjects who had undergone Nd:YAG LPI for uveitis due to iris bombe. Twenty-eight (28) LPIs were performed, 17 of which resulted in failure [24]. The same study noted that among 99 patients with no history of uveitis, there were no instances of LPI failure. Meanwhile, for eyes with no active inflammation at the time of LPI as well as those showing severe inflammatory reaction at the time of LPI, the failure rates were comparable: 40–60%. Agraval et al. proposed a mathematical model for the determination of the optimal iridectomy size in uveitic eyes. Based on this model, and in consideration of increased aqueous viscosity and atrophic/floppy iris in uveitic eyes, a minimum LPI diameter of 300–350 microns was recommended [25].

Pigment dispersion syndrome is considered to be a predisposing factor for the development of pigmentary glaucoma [26]. The mechanism leading to pigment deposition in anterior-segment structures entails rubbing of the surface of the posterior iris against the lens zonules, which occurs due to posterior bowing of the concave iris root [27, 28]. LPI can reduce this "reverse pupillary block" by establishing an anterior-/posterior-chamber pressure balance [29, 30]. However, whether LPI-induced reduction of posterior bowing of the iris alters disease courses is debated still. Gandolfi et al. conducted a 10-year follow-up study on pigment dispersion syndrome eyes, reporting that LPI can reduce IOP elevation rates in eyes at high risk of progression to glaucoma [31]. In a randomized trial involving a 3-year follow-up, though, LPI's effect in preventing pigment dispersion syndrome progression to pigmentary glaucoma was unclear [32]. Michelessi and Lindsley likewise concluded that the evidence on LPI's putative role in preventing or reducing glaucoma progression is inconclusive and insufficient, they and two other studies having noted flatter irises but no significant IOP reduction [33–35].

5.3 Performing Laser Peripheral Iridotomy

5.3.1 Choice of Laser and Laser Settings

Head-to-head trials that have compared argon with Nd:YAG laser iridotomy indicate the efficacy of the Nd:YAG laser. Several studies on mainly Caucasian populations have shown more frequent closure for argon laser iridotomies [36–38]. Del Priore in fact found no closure in any eyes receiving Nd:YAG iridotomy over the course of follow-up periods covering 20–42 months, whereas 21% of the same patients' contralateral eyes that had been treated by argon laser required retreatment for iridotomy closure [37]. Also, Nd:YAG iridotomy requires far fewer laser applications and less laser energy, enabling a faster and more easily tolerated procedure (Fig. 5.2) [37, 38].

The rates of most short-term complications (e.g., nonprogressive corneal opacification; IOP spikes) are similar between the two lasers [36, 38]. Hyphemas, however, occur with more frequency (≥30%) in Nd:YAG-treated eyes, and only rarely in cases of argon laser use [37, 38]. Hyphema rates can be reduced by pre-treating Nd:YAG LPI patients using the argon laser at the intended site of iridotomy. In one study, argon-pretreated eyes showed a 17% bleeding rate compared with a 67% rate for eyes treated with Nd:YAG alone [39]. The combination of these two lasers also enables iris perforation with a smaller number of Nd:YAG pulses, especially for patients with dark irises [40], and is a commonly employed modality in some regions of Asia.

In the case of argon laser iridotomy, the typical settings are as follows: spot size, 50 microns; power, 500–1000 mW; duration, 0.02–0.2 seconds. For Nd:YAG laser iridotomy meanwhile, energy levels ranging between 2 and 10 mJ are required. In studies on primarily Caucasian populations, the total energies necessary for argon laser iridotomy have averaged between 10 and 20 J, whereas those for Nd:YAG laser iridotomy have fallen within the 30–40 mJ range [36, 38]. For darker-iris populations, significantly higher Nd:YAG laser energy might be required, as has been reported based on a large case series of patients treated in the Kingdom of Saudi Arabia: over 100 mJ, on average, for Nd:YAG LPI [1]. The energy required for Nd:YAG LPI can be still higher in cases of acute angle closure (AAC): one study from Saudi Arabia recorded a 152 mJ average for AAC eyes relative to 123 and 98 mJ means for eyes with occludable angles and chronic angle-closure, respectively [1].

5.3.2 Laser Techniques

A laser is most efficaciously applied through focusing lenses such as a 66 diopters (D) Abraham lens or a 103 D Wise lens, which enable the application of energy directly to the iris surface, increasing of power applied per pulse, and decreasing of the exposure of other tissues such as the cornea, lens, or retina [41]. Laser energy ideally is applied to the superior iris such that the iridotomy site is covered by the upper eyelid. The iridotomy should be as peripheral as is possible, though in cases of peripheral corneal opacities (e.g., arcus senilis) or iris–cornea apposition, iridotomies that are less peripheral might be necessary.

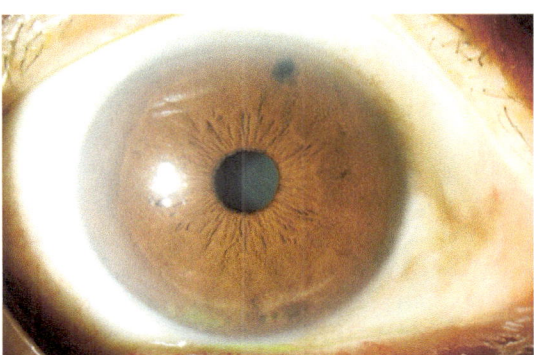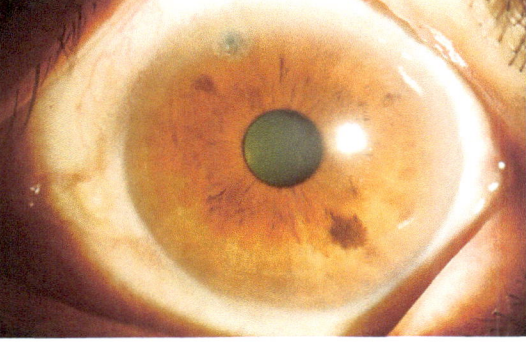

Fig. 5.2 Anterior segment photograph after argon (left) and Nd:YAG (right) laser peripheral iridotomy

As the iridotomy site, either an iris crypt or an area of thinning or atrophy should be chosen in order to minimize the energy that is necessary to form a patent hole. Placement exactly at 12 o'clock is discouraged, because air bubbles generated during the procedure (as is typical when employing the argon laser) generally accumulate there, with the result that the clinician's view is obscured [42].

Iris perforation often is accompanied by a flood of fluid, with iris epithelium pigment, into the anterior chamber. At this point, further laser application for iridotomy enlargement usually is desired, but, due to either the reason just noted or corneal clouding, the view of the iris might be limited. Waiting for settling of pigment, or having the patient return for a subsequent visit, can facilitate treatment in such a way that does not subject him to gratuitously large amounts of laser energy. Because laser application through the iridotomy site is potentially injurious to the lens, retina, or fovea, care should be exercised to focus on the remaining iris tissue once the patent hole is formed [43–46].

LPI can be used as an adjunct with Argon laser peripheral iridoplasty (ALPI). Park et al. reported that ALPI combined LPI therapy had a much greater effect of anterior chamber angle widening compared with LPI alone [47].

5.3.3 Pre- and Post-laser Medications

Fifteen to sixty minutes before the iridotomy, eyes can be treated with pilocarpine (1–4%) in order to obtain miosis and thin the iris. At the same time, topical apraclonidine should be applied for the prevention of postoperative pressure spikes [48, 49], though other pressure-lowering agents (e.g., brimonidine, dorzolamide) also can be effective [50, 51]. Apraclonidine, thanks to its vasoconstrictive efficacy, might also reduce the hyphema risk. Pressure spike absence should be confirmed by IOP check 1–2 h following the procedure. Post treatment, patients are administered topical steroid to reduce inflammation. The steroid dose needs to be increased in eyes showing active inflammation at LPI or those with a history of uveitis.

5.4 Results of Laser Peripheral Iridotomy

5.4.1 Acute Angle Closure

Long-term post-LPI control of IOP for AAC cases frequently is a problem, most relevant studies having shown a need for supplemental IOP lowering treatment months or years after LPI. In a Singaporean study, 58% of patients after a mean follow-up of more than 4 years required such treatment notwithstanding patent LPI obtainment; included in this number were 32% who had gone on to trabeculectomy [2]. Another Singapore-based study showed comparable results: 41% of patients underwent additional treatment within 1 year due to an IOP rise above 21 mmHg [4]. Two other studies, these from the UK, similarly found that more than half of AAC patients required post-LPI treatment. Choong reported, after a 6-month follow-up period, that 56% of eyes needed supplemental treatment, including 25% that required a surgical procedure [52]. Saunders found that 63% underwent treatment within 8 months, including 41% who required surgery [3]. Eyes that would subsequently require additional pressure-lowering treatment had begun with more peripheral anterior synechiae (PAS) and narrower angles than had eyes not needing any additional treatment [4]. Hsiao in Taiwan noted a stronger impact of pre-LPI PAS, 83% of eyes going on to trabeculectomy having shown greater than 270 degrees of pre-LPI PAS [5]. Thus, close monitoring of IOP is advised in following up on AAC patients, even after LPI has been successfully performed.

Choi et al. reported that 32% of eyes manifested PAS progression over the course of a 3-year post-LPI follow-up. The PAS progression risk was higher in eyes with plateau iris as well as in eyes that had proved, before LPI, relatively unresponsive to medication [53]. Changes in angle width also have been evaluated using ASOCT. An Iran-based study, for example, showed that in AAC eyes, LPI had resulted in significantly increased angle width, anterior-chamber depth, anterior-chamber area, and iris flattening [54].

5.4.2 Chronic Angle-Closure Glaucoma

Several studies on PACG patients of various ethnic backgrounds have noted both short- and long-term IOP lowering after LPI [1, 5–11]. A total of 187 Saudi Arabian PACG eyes showed a significant mean-IOP drop from 24.8 to 17.5 mmHg, equal numbers of patients having received medical therapy 12 months after LPI [1]. A mostly Caucasian population that had been treated with argon LPI for PACG and followed for 53 months showed a mean IOP decrease from 28 to 18.5 mmHg and a medication-number decrease from 1.5 to 0.9 [10]. It should be noted, however, that 10 of the 98 eyes treated required trabeculectomy at some point during the follow-up period. A study on 58 Taiwanese PACG eyes reported a mean IOP decrease from 25.4 to 14.1 mmHg over the course of a mean 51-month follow-up period [5]. All but 7% of those eyes required either the same number or fewer medicines to reach this lower pressure, though almost half remained on some form of medical therapy at the end of the follow-up, while 4 of the 58 eyes (7%) required trabeculectomy.

Other studies have reported substantially higher post-LPI trabeculectomy rates for PACG [55]. Richardson and Cooper found that 62% of PACG cases with field loss needed additional treatment (i.e., increasing strength/number of drops, laser, and/or trabeculectomy) by an average of 15.3 months post-LPI. By contrast, only 31% of PACG cases without field loss required more treatment, and only 1 of those eyes needed

trabeculectomy [9]. Nolan et al., having evaluated 164 Mongolian eyes in cases of angle-closure disease, reported rates of treatment failure (i.e., requiring surgery for control of IOP, or an acuity drop to less than 3/60): 48% of eyes that had shown glaucomatous optic neuropathy at the baseline failed, whereas only 3% of those not showing glaucomatous optic neuropathy did so [55].

Therefore, it should be noted that in patients with PACG, additional medicine and surgery can be required in the long-term disease progression even after successful LPI.

5.4.3 Primary Angle Closure and Primary Angle-Closure Suspect

The studies reporting on IOP control of LPI in cases of PAC/PACS are summarized in Table 5.2. Three studies including a combined total of 153 PACS eyes all reported no IOP increases over a mean follow-up period ranging from 11 to 46 months [8, 56, 57]. Peng et al. evaluated long-term LPI outcomes for 239 PACS eyes. IOP elevation greater than 21 mmHg was evident in 18% of eyes after a mean follow-up interval of 56 months, 7% needed further treatment, and 0.4% needed glaucoma surgery [58].

Sihota et al. evaluated IOP responses to various provocative tests both before and 1 month following LPI in 50 PAC eyes showing PAS but no IOP elevation [59]. A positive result was deemed to be an IOP increase of 6 mmHg or more from the baseline. Meanwhile, the mydriatic-provocative positivity rate, for example, was found to have decreased from 26 to 15% after LPI. In another three retrospective studies on PAC eyes, further, post-LPI treatment was required in 42–67% of cases over the course of a follow-up duration of 46 months to 12 years [57, 58, 60]. Further treatment after LPI mainly entailed medical therapy, relatively few patients having required glaucoma surgery (0–13%).

Table 5.2 Intraocular pressure control of LPI in cases of PAC or PACS

Study (year)	Race	Number of eyes	Angle	Duration	IOP elevation	Progression
Nolan (2000)	Mongolian	PACS 74	ITC ≥ 270	11 and 35 months (2 groups)	0	0
Pandav (2007)	Indian	PACS 27	ITC ≥ 180	45.6 months	0	0
		PAC 43			83.7% > 21 mmHg	9.3% to PACG
Ramani (2009)	Indian	PACS 52	ITC ≥ 180	2 years	0	29% to PAC
Peng (2011)	Vietnamese	PACS 239	ITC ≥ 180	11.8 years	85.5% > 21 mmHg	22.2% to PAC, 3.8% to PACG
		PAC 99				5.2% to PACG
Rao (2013)	Indian	PAC 16	ITC ≥ 180	50 months		0

LPI laser peripheral iridotomy, *PAC* primary angle closure, *PACS* primary angle-closure suspect, *ITC* iridotrabecular contact, *PACG* primary angle-closure glaucoma

5.5 Complications of Laser Peripheral Iridotomy

5.5.1 Intraocular Pressure Spikes

In the early years of LPI, transient pressure spikes represented a significant problem [61], but ever since the availability of apraclonidine for prevention of post-LPI pressure spikes, they are much less common [49]. Robin et al. showed that, among 14 eyes treated with apraclonidine prior to argon LPI, none experienced any IOP rise greater than 10 mmHg following the procedure, which compared favorably with 14 placebo-treated eyes, 6 of which experienced IOP rise. Among Japanese eyes treated by Nd:YAG iridotomy, only 1 of 29 treated with preoperative apraclonidine manifested a pressure rise of 10 mmHg or greater, as compared with 5 of 29 of eyes that had not received preoperative apraclonidine [62]. In another study, this one on 289 eyes lacking any significant glaucomatous optic neuropathy, only 2 treated preoperatively with apraclonidine showed pressure increases of 10 mmHg or more, which in fact suggests that IOP monitoring after routine LPI might be less necessary than previously thought [48]. Other topical pressure-lowering agents such as dorzolamide and brimonidine have demonstrated similar effectiveness for prevention of post-LPI spikes in IOP. Thus, other medications may be substituted in cases where apraclonidine is unavailable [50, 51].

5.5.2 Cataract Progression

Several studies have estimated post-LPI cataract progression risk. Lim et al. found that post-LPI cataract progression occurred in as many as 23% of 60 fellow AAC eyes [43], and Tan et al. noted 38% progression among 42 AAC eyes [63]. These studies' follow-up durations were 27 and 12 months, respectively, and in both cases, cataract progression was defined as 2 or more units of increase, in any lens region, in Lens Opacities Classification System II or III grading. However, neither study used a control group, and as such, natural cataract progression in such eyes was not determined. Vijaya et al. compared 6-years-post-LPI cataract progression in 190 PACS eyes with a 3015-subject control group that had not undergone LPI [64]. They defined cataract progression as either 2 or more units of change on the Lens Opacities Classification System II scale or a history of cataract surgery in the baseline/follow-up examination interval. The cataract progression risk was significantly higher in the post-LPI subjects (odds ratio, 1.7): progression occurred in 39% of LPI cases versus 23% of non-LPI cases.

Cases of Nd:YAG LPI lens rupture leading to either anterior-chamber cortical material or sterile granulomatous endophthalmitis have been reported [65, 66]. Moreover, LPI has been found to result in iris flattening and increased iris lens contact resulting most likely from aqueous flow redirection [67]. Increased iris-lens contact or redirected aqueous humor flow potentially will result in cataractous change.

5.5.3 Change in Endothelial Cell Count

Kumar et al. compared endothelial cell density in 230 post-LPI PACS eyes with that in untreated fellow eyes in a prospective study. They found that the endothelial cell density had decreased from the baseline to post-LPI 3 years in both the treated (2%) and the fellow (0.9%) eyes, but that this did not represent a statistically significant difference [68]. Another retrospective study evaluated endothelial cell count changes in AAC eyes that had been treated with either LPI (32 eyes) or phacoemulsification (16 eyes). In both groups, the endothelial cell count had decreased continuously from the baseline. At the 24-month follow-ups, however, the LPI group showed significantly higher endothelial cell count loss than did the phacoemulsification group (23 vs. 13%) [69]. This diminished endothelial cell count in AAC eyes was, as would be expected, higher than among PACS subjects in the above-noted study [68].

5.5.4 Anterior-Chamber Bleeding

Bleeding has been reported in up to 67% of eyes having undergone Nd:YAG LPI [37–39]. Bleeding with argon iridotomy is comparatively rare, and argon laser pretreatment of the iridotomy site prior to Nd:YAG iridotomy can minimize bleeding [39]. Ahmadi et al. reported a higher frequency of hyphema occurrence in cases of superior LPI (41%) relative to inferior LPI (30%), which difference was statistically significant [70]. Vera et al., meanwhile, having compared intraoperative bleeding incidence between cases of superior and temporal LPI, found no difference (9 vs. 10%) [71].

Golan et al. evaluated prospectively the effect of antithrombotic medications (i.e., aspirin, warfarin, clopidogrel) on anterior-chamber bleeding. Two hundred and eight (208) PACS subjects underwent right-eye LPI while continuing with antithrombotic medications, the left eye undergoing LPI 2 weeks after discontinuation of the medication [72]. The incidence of severe bleeding was similar, whether the patient was on or off the medications. There was a significant right/left-eye correlation between bleeders in that most who bled from the right (on medication) eye also bled from the left (off medication) eye. These results indicate strongly that antithrombotic medication does not need to be discontinued prior to LPI, and that specific patients might have a tendency to bleed regardless of being on or off of medication.

5.5.5 Dysphotopsia

Patients with patent iridotomies might have dysphotopsias such as holes, blurred horizontal line, ghost images, glare, shadows, and so forth [73–75]. Vera et al. conducted a comparative trial that was randomized and single-masked as well as paired-eye in order to assess the LPI-location effect on dysphotopsia occurrence. A total of 169 PAC/PACS patients who had been randomized to receive LPI either temporally in 1 eye or superiorly in the other were analyzed. Both LPIs had been performed, sequentially, on the same day, and a questionnaire inquiring of any symptoms of visual disturbance was completed within 1 month of LPI. New-onset linear dysphotopsia was significantly more reported for eyes with superior LPIs (11%) than for those with temporal LPIs (2%) [71]. They indicated redirection of the light through the tear meniscus of the upper lid can be the cause of symptoms. Congdon et al. assessed LPI's impact on subjective visual symptoms and forward-scattering of light based on the measurement of retinal stray light. In both cases, there was no difference between the 217 post-LPI PACS subjects and 250 age- and gender-matched controls. Glare prevalence did not differ with LPI location with respect to the eyelid. However, it should be noted that this randomized trial's results could have been affected by the relatively long duration—18 months—between LPI and glare evaluation [76]. In a multicenter prospective trial, the frequency of any symptoms of new-onset dysphotopsia was compared between 559 patients who had been randomized for either bilateral superior or bilateral nasal/temporal LPI. According to a multivariate logistic regression analysis, neither LPI location, LPI area, nor total laser energy predicted a higher probability of new postoperative dysphotopsia [77].

5.5.6 Other Complications

Inflammation after LPI has been reported in two studies: the EAGLE study reported that in 0.5% of eyes (1/211), post-LPI inflammation was shown, though neither severity nor duration of inflammation was specified [78]; in the other study, 69% of PACG eyes showed grade 2+ or higher uveitis after LPI treatment, though most of the cases were resolved within 48–72 h of treatment with topical corticosteroid [70]. A case of foveal photocoagulation has been reported for a patient who had undergone argon laser iridotomy with the Abraham contact lens [46]. Visual acuity decreased ultimately to 20/400, and a visible foveal RPE depigmentation area was shown.

Compliance with Ethical Requirements
Conflict of interest: Young Kook Kim and Ki Ho Park declare that they have no conflict of interest.
Informed consent: No human studies were carried out by the authors for this chapter.
Animal studies: No animal studies were carried out by the authors for this chapter.

References

1. Tomey K, Traverso C, Shammas I. Neodymium-YAG laser iridotomy in the treatment and prevention of angle closure glaucoma. A review of 373 eyes. Arch Ophthalmol. 1987;105:476–81.
2. Aung T, Ang LP, Chan S-P, Chew PT. Acute primary angle-closure: long-term intraocular pressure outcome in Asian eyes. Am J Ophthalmol. 2001;131:7–12.
3. Saunders D. Acute closed-angle glaucoma and Nd-YAG laser iridotomy. Br J Ophthalmol. 1990;74:523–5.
4. Lim LS, Aung T, Husain R, et al. Acute primary angle closure: configuration of the drainage angle in the first year after laser peripheral iridotomy. Ophthalmology. 2004;111:1470–4.
5. Hsiao C-H, Hsu C-T, Shen S-C, Chen HS. Mid-term follow-up of Nd: YAG laser iridotomy in Asian eyes. Ophthalmic Surg Lasers Imaging Retina. 2003;34:291.
6. Langerhorst CT, Kluyver EB, van den Berg TJ. Effect of peripheral iridectomy on intraocular pressure in chronic primary angle closure glaucoma. Doc Ophthalmol. 1993;85:51–4.
7. McGalliard JN, Wishart PK. The effect of Nd:YAG iridotomy on intraocular pressure in hypertensive eyes with shallow anterior chambers. Eye. 1990;4(Pt 6):823–9.
8. Nolan WP, Foster PJ, Devereux JG, et al. YAG laser iridotomy treatment for primary angle closure in east Asian eyes. Br J Ophthalmol. 2000;84:1255–9.
9. Richardson P, Cooper RL. Laser iridotomy. Aust N Z J Ophthalmol. 1987;15:119–23.
10. Robin AL, Pollack IP. Argon laser peripheral iridotomies in the treatment of primary angle closure glaucoma. Long-term follow-up. Arch Ophthalmol. 1982;100:919–23.
11. Salmon JF. Long-term intraocular pressure control after Nd-YAG laser Iridotomy in chronic angle-closure Glaucoma. J Glaucoma. 1993;2:291–6.
12. Jiang Y, Chang DS, Zhu H, et al. Longitudinal changes of angle configuration in primary angle-closure suspects: the Zhongshan angle-closure prevention trial. Ophthalmology. 2014;121:1699–705.
13. Lee KS, Sung KR, Shon K, et al. Longitudinal changes in anterior segment parameters after laser peripheral iridotomy assessed by anterior segment optical coherence tomography. Invest Ophthalmol Vis Sci. 2013;54:3166–70.
14. Anderson DR, Forster RK, Lewis ML. Laser iridotomy for aphakic pupillary block. Arch Ophthalmol. 1975;93:343–6.
15. Weinberger D, Lusky M, Debbi S, Ben-Sira I. Pseudophakic and aphakic pupillary block. Ann Ophthalmol. 1988;20:403–5.
16. Werner D, Kaback M. Pseudophakic pupillary-block glaucoma. Br J Ophthalmol. 1977;61:329–33.
17. Cinotti DJ, Maltzman BA, Reiter DJ, Cinotti AA. Neodymium:YAG laser therapy for pseudophakic pupillary block. J Cataract Refract Surg. 1986;12:174–9.
18. Khokhar S, Sethi HS, Sony P, et al. Pseudophakic pupillary block caused by pupillary capture after phacoemulsification and in-the-bag AcrySof lens implantation. J Cataract Refract Surg. 2002;28:1291–2.
19. Naveh N, Wysenbeek Y, Solomon A, et al. Anterior capsule adherence to iris leading to pseudophakic pupillary block. Ophthalmic Surg. 1991;22:350–2.
20. Vajpayee RB, Angra SK, Titiyal JS, et al. Pseudophakic pupillary-block glaucoma in children. Am J Ophthalmol. 1991;111:715–8.

21. Kokoris N, Macy JI. Laser iridectomy treatment of acute pseudophakic pupillary block glaucoma. J Am Intraocul Implant Soc. 1982;8:33–4.
22. Gaton D, Mimouni K, Lusky M, et al. Pupillary block following posterior chamber intraocular lens implantation in adults. Br J Ophthalmol. 2003;87:1109–11.
23. Shrader CE, Belcher CD 3rd, Thomas JV, et al. Pupillary and iridovitreal block in pseudophakic eyes. Ophthalmology. 1984;91:831–7.
24. Karickhoff JR. Pigmentary dispersion syndrome and pigmentary glaucoma: a new mechanism concept, a new treatment, and a new technique. Ophthalmic Surg. 1992;23:269–77.
25. Spencer NA, Hall AJ, Stawell RJ. Nd:YAG laser iridotomy in uveitic glaucoma. Clin Exp Ophthalmol. 2001;29:217–9.
26. Agraval U, Qi N, Stewart P, et al. Optimum size of iridotomy in uveitis. Clin Exp Ophthalmol. 2015;43:692–6.
27. Richter CU, Richardson TM, Grant WM. Pigmentary dispersion syndrome and pigmentary glaucoma. A prospective study of the natural history. Arch Ophthalmol. 1986;104:211–5.
28. Campbell DG. Pigmentary dispersion and glaucoma. A new theory. Arch Ophthalmol. 1979;97:1667–72.
29. Scuderi G, Nucci C, Palma S, Cerulli L. Iris configuration in pigment dispersion syndrome: effects of miotics and YAG laser peripheral iridotomy. Invest Ophthalmol Vis Sci: LIPPINCOTT-RAVEN PUBL, PA 19106, 1997; v. 38.
30. Chen M, Lin S. Effect of a YAG laser iridotomy on intraocular pressure in pigmentary glaucoma. Br J Ophthalmol. 2002;86:1443–4.
31. Gandolfi SA, Ungaro N, Tardini MG, et al. A 10-year follow-up to determine the effect of YAG laser iridotomy on the natural history of pigment dispersion syndrome: a randomized clinical trial. JAMA ophthalmol. 2014;132:1433–8.
32. Scott A, Kotecha A, Bunce C, et al. YAG laser peripheral iridotomy for the prevention of pigment dispersion glaucoma: a prospective, randomized, controlled trial. Ophthalmology. 2011;118:468–73.
33. Michelessi M, Lindsley K. Peripheral iridotomy for pigmentary glaucoma. Cochrane Database Syst Rev. 2016;(2):CD005655. https://doi.org/10.1002/14651858.CD005655.pub2.
34. Costa V, Gandham S, Spaeth G, et al. The effect of nd-yag laser iridotomy on pigmentary glaucoma patients-a prospective-study. Invest Ophthalmol Vis Sci: Lippincott-Raven PUBL 227 EAST WASHINGTON SQ, PHILADELPHIA, PA 19106, 1994; v. 35.
35. Georgopoulos G, Papaconstantinou D, Patsea L, et al. Laser iridotomy versus low dose pilocarpine treatment in patients with pigmentary glaucoma. Invest Ophthalmol Vis Sci: Assoc Research Vision Ophthalmology Inc 9650 ROCKVILLE PIKE, 2001; v. 42.
36. Robin AL, Pollack IP. A comparison of neodymium: YAG end argon laser Iridotomies. Ophthalmology. 1984;91:1011–6.
37. Del Priore LV, Robin AL, Pollack IP. Neodymium: YAG and argon laser iridotomy: long-term follow-up in a prospective, randomized clinical trial. Ophthalmology. 1988;95:1207–11.
38. Moster MR, Schwartz LW, Spaeth GL, et al. Laser iridectomy: a controlled study comparing argon and neodymium: YAG. Ophthalmology. 1986;93:20–4.
39. Goins K, Schmeisser E, Smith T. Argon laser pretreatment in Nd: YAG iridotomy. Ophthalmic Surg Lasers Imaging Retina. 1990;21:497–500.
40. Ho T, Fan R. Sequential argon-YAG laser iridotomies in dark irides. Br J Ophthalmol. 1992;76:329–31.
41. Wise JB, Munnerlyn CR, Erickson PJ. A high-efficiency laser iridotomy-sphincterctomy lens. Am J Ophthalmol. 1986;101:546–53.
42. Quigley HA. Long-term follow-up of laser iridotomy. Ophthalmology. 1981;88:218–24.
43. Lim LS, Husain R, Gazzard G, et al. Cataract progression after prophylactic laser peripheral iridotomy: potential implications for the prevention of glaucoma blindness. Ophthalmology. 2005;112:1355–9.
44. Welch DB, Apple DJ, Mendelsohn AD, et al. Lens injury following iridotomy with a Q-switched neodymium-YAG laser. Arch Ophthalmol. 1986;104:123–5.
45. Bongard B, Pederson JE. Retinal burns from experimental laser iridotomy. Ophthalmic Surg Lasers Imaging Retina. 1985;16:42–4.
46. Berger BB. Foveal photocoagulation from laser iridotomy. Ophthalmology. 1984;91:1029–33.
47. Park HJ, Park KH, Kim SH, et al. Change in angle parameters measured by anterior segment optical coherence tomography after laser peripheral Iridotomy alone versus laser peripheral Iridotomy and argon laser peripheral Iridoplasty. J Korean Ophthalmol Soc. 2011;52:566–73.
48. Lewis R, Perkins TW, Gangnon R, et al. The rarity of clinically significant rise in intraocular pressure after laser peripheral iridotomy with apraclonidine. Ophthalmology. 1998;105:2256–9.
49. Robin AL, Pollack IP. Effects of topical ALO 2145 (p-aminoclonidine hydrochloride) on the acute intraocular pressure rise after argon laser iridotomy. Arch Ophthalmol. 1987;105:1208–11.
50. Chen TC. Brimonidine 0.15% versus apraclonidine 0.5% for prevention of intraocular pressure elevation after anterior segment laser surgery. J Cataract Refract Surg. 2005;31:1707–12.
51. Hartenbaum D, Wilson H, Maloney S, et al. A randomized study of dorzolamide in the prevention of elevated intraocular pressure after anterior segment laser surgery. Dorzolamide laser study group. J Glaucoma. 1999;8:273–5.
52. Choong YF, Irfan S, Menage MJ. Acute angle closure glaucoma: an evaluation of a protocol for acute treatment. Eye. 1999;13(Pt 5):613–6.
53. Choi JS, Kim YY. Progression of peripheral anterior synechiae after laser iridotomy. Am J Ophthalmol. 2005;140:1125–7.

54. Moghimi S, Chen R, Johari M, et al. Changes in anterior segment morphology after laser peripheral Iridotomy in acute primary angle closure. Am J Ophthalmol. 2016;166:133–40.
55. Nolan W. Lens extraction in primary angle closure. Br J Ophthalmol. 2006;90:1–2.
56. Ramani KK, Mani B, George RJ, Lingam V. Follow-up of primary angle closure suspects after laser peripheral iridotomy using ultrasound biomicroscopy and A-scan biometry for a period of 2 years. J Glaucoma. 2009;18:521–7.
57. Pandav SS, Kaushik S, Jain R, et al. Laser peripheral iridotomy across the spectrum of primary angle closure. Can J Ophthalmol. 2007;42:233–7.
58. Peng P-H, Nguyen H, Lin H-S, et al. Long-term outcomes of laser iridotomy in Vietnamese patients with primary angle closure. Br J Ophthalmol. 2011;95:1207–11.
59. Sihota R, Rishi K, Srinivasan G, et al. Functional evaluation of an iridotomy in primary angle closure eyes. Graefes Arch Clin Exp Ophthalmol. 2016;254:1141–9.
60. Rao A, Rao HL, Kumar AU, et al. Outcomes of laser peripheral iridotomy in angle closure disease. Semin Ophthalmol. 2013;28:4–8.
61. Krupin T, Stone RA, Cohen BH, et al. Acute intraocular pressure response to argon laser iridotomy. Ophthalmology. 1985;92:922–6.
62. Kitazawa Y, Taniguchi T, Sugiyama K. Use of apraclonidine to reduce acute intraocular pressure rise following Q-switched Nd:YAG laser iridotomy. Ophthalmic Surg. 1989;20:49–52.
63. Tan AM, Loon SC, Chew PT. Outcomes following acute primary angle closure in an Asian population. Clin Exp Ophthalmol. 2009;37:467–72.
64. Vijaya L, Asokan R, Panday M, George R. Is prophylactic laser peripheral iridotomy for primary angle closure suspects a risk factor for cataract progression? The Chennai eye disease incidence study. Br J Ophthalmol. 2017;101:665–70.
65. Fernandez-Bahamonde J. Iatrogenic lens rupture after a neodymium: yttrium aluminum garnet laser iridotomy attempt. Ann Ophthalmol. 1991;23:346–8.
66. Margo CE, Lessner A, Goldey SH, Sherwood M. Lens-induced endophthalmitis after Nd:YAG laser iridotomy. Am J Ophthalmol. 1992;113:97–8.
67. Caronia RM, Liebmann JM, Stegman Z, et al. Increase in iris-lens contact after laser iridotomy for pupillary block angle closure. Am J Ophthalmol. 1996;122:53–7.
68. Kumar RS, Baskaran M, Friedman DS, et al. Effect of prophylactic laser iridotomy on corneal endothelial cell density over 3 years in primary angle closure suspects. Br J Ophthalmol. 2013;97:258–61.
69. Park HY, Lee NY, Park CK, Kim MS. Long-term changes in endothelial cell counts after early phacoemulsification versus laser peripheral iridotomy using sequential argon:YAG laser technique in acute primary angle closure. Graefes Arch Clin Exp Ophthalmol. 2012;250:1673–80.
70. Ahmadi M, Naderi Beni Z, Naderi Beni A, Kianersi F. Efficacy of neodymium-doped yttrium aluminum garnet laser iridotomies in primary angle-closure diseases: superior peripheral iridotomy versus inferior peripheral iridotomy. Curr Med Res Opin. 2017;33:687–92.
71. Vera V, Naqi A, Belovay GW, et al. Dysphotopsia after temporal versus superior laser peripheral iridotomy: a prospective randomized paired eye trial. Am J Ophthalmol. 2014;157:929–935.e922.
72. Golan S, Levkovitch-Verbin H, Shemesh G, Kurtz S. Anterior chamber bleeding after laser peripheral iridotomy. JAMA Ophthalmol. 2013;131:626–9.
73. Murphy PH, Trope GE. Monocular blurring. A complication of YAG laser iridotomy. Ophthalmology. 1991;98:1539–42.
74. Chung RSH, Guan AEK. Unusual visual disturbance following laser peripheral iridotomy for intermittent angle closure glaucoma. Graefes Arch Clin Exp Ophthalmol. 2006;244:532–3.
75. Weintraub J, Berke SJ. Blurring after iridotomy. Ophthalmology. 1992;99:479–80.
76. Congdon N, Yan X, Friedman DS, et al. Visual symptoms and retinal straylight after laser peripheral iridotomy: the Zhongshan angle-closure prevention trial. Ophthalmology. 2012;119:1375–82.
77. Srinivasan K, Zebardast N, Krishnamurthy P, et al. Comparison of new visual disturbances after superior versus nasal/temporal laser peripheral iridotomy: a prospective randomized trial. Ophthalmology. 2018;125:345–51.
78. Azuara-Blanco A, Burr J, Ramsay C, et al. Effectiveness of early lens extraction for the treatment of primary angle-closure glaucoma (EAGLE): a randomised controlled trial. Lancet. 2016;388:1389–97.

Laser Peripheral Iridoplasty

6

Robert Ritch and Clement C. Y. Tham

Abstracts

Argon Laser Peripheral Iridoplasty (ALPI) opens up appositionally-closed portions of the anterior chamber drainage angle with low-power, larger-spot-size, longer-duration laser contraction applications on the far periphery of the iris. The laser applications induce contraction and thinning of the iris stroma, and thereby open up the space between the iris and the trabecular meshwork.

ALPI is indicated in primary angle closure disease (PACD), in particular primary angle closure (PAC) and primary angle closure glaucoma (PACG). ALPI is effective and safe in aborting acute angle closure, bcth primary and certain forms of secondary types. It is also useful in other situations wher. ocular hypertension is caused by more extensive appositional angle closure.

In this chapter, the techniques of ALPI are described. The complications of ALPI, their avoidance and management, are discussed. Surgical tips and pearls in performing ALPI, and how to make ALPI a safe and effective option in the management of angle closure, are presented.

Keywords

Argon laser peripheral iridoplasty · ALPI · Angle closure · Glaucoma

R. Ritch
Einhorn Clinical Research Center, The New York Eye and Ear Infirmary of Mount Sinai, New York, NY, USA

Founder, Secretary and Chairman, Scientific Advisory Board, The Glaucoma Foundation, New York, NY, USA
e-mail: ritchmd@glaucoma.net

C. C. Y. Tham (✉)
Department of Ophthalmology and Visual Sciences, The Chinese University of Hong Kong, Hong Kong, SAR, China

Prince of Wales Hospital, Shatin, Hong Kong, SAR, China

Hong Kong Eye Hospital, Kowloon, Hong Kong, SAR, China

Department of Ophthalmology and Visual Sciences, The Chinese University of Hong Kong, Hong Kong Eye Hospital, Hong Kong, SAR, China
e-mail: clemtham@cuhk.edu.hk

6.1 The Concept and Uses of Argon Laser Peripheral Iridoplasty (ALPI)

Argon laser peripheral iridoplasty (ALPI) is a simple and effective procedure in opening an appositionally closed angle in situations in which laser iridotomy (LI) cannot be pe:formed or that there is persistent appositional clcsure despite LI due to the presence of mechanisms other than pupillary block. The procedure consists of inducing contraction burns (low power. long duration, and large spot size) to the peripheral iris in order

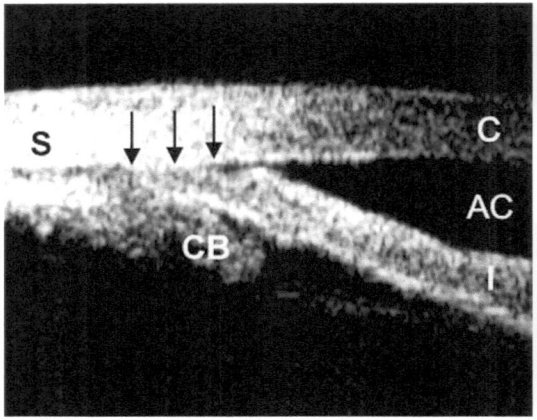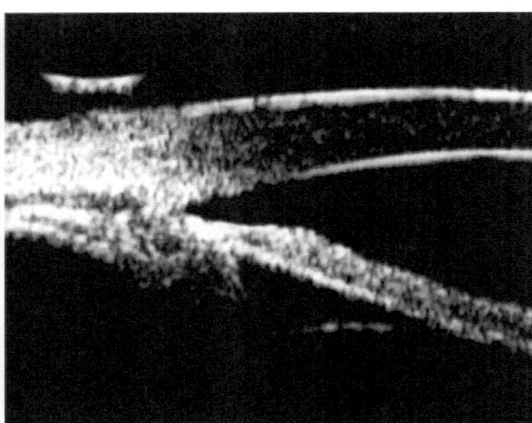

Fig. 6.1 Ultrasound biomicroscopic (UBM) images illustrating how ALPI contracts the peripheral iris stroma, creating a space between the anterior iris surface and the trabecular meshwork, thus opening the angle. Left: appositionally closed angle in an eye with plateau iris syndrome. Right: open angle after ALPI

to physically pull and open up the angle via contraction of iris stroma at the site of burn (Fig. 6.1) [1–5]. ALPI is useful in reversing an attack of acute angle closure (AAC), either as an immediate initial approach to treatment or when glaucoma medications fail to break the attack. The diagnostic indications for ALPI require the ability of the ophthalmologist to differentiate subtle gonioscopic findings. The examiner must be facile with darkroom indentation gonioscopy and with the anatomic causes of angle closure and the means of diagnosing these clinically [6].

6.2   History and Developments

Krasnov [7] was the first to attempt to use laser burns near the iris root to separate iris and trabecular meshwork. The initial procedure encompassed only 90° of the angle. The laser parameters used in these early attempts were more like penetrating burns than the slow contraction burns which later proved optimal, and were often unsuccessful because of insufficient retraction of the iris from the meshwork. Kimbrough et al. [8] described a technique for direct treatment of 360° of the peripheral iris through a gonioscopy lens,

and termed the procedure *gonioplasty*. The modern technique of argon laser peripheral iridoplasty was initially described for breaking medically unresponsive attacks of acute angle closure [1]. The history, indications, techniques, and results of the procedure up to a decade ago were extensively reviewed [9].

6.3   Indications for ALPI and outcomes

6.3.1   Primary Angle Closure Glaucoma: Acute and Chronic

6.3.1.1 Acute Angle Closure
Laser peripheral iridotomy (LPI) is the definitive treatment for acute angle closure in order to eliminate any component of pupillary block, even if other mechanisms are present or predominate. An attack of AAC that is unresponsive to medical therapy and in which corneal edema, a shallow anterior chamber, or marked inflammation precludes immediate iridotomy, or an attack which is unresponsive despite successful iris penetration by iridotomy, may be broken with ALPI [1, 10–13]. Circumferential treatment of the iris

opens the angle in those areas in which there are no peripheral anterior synechiae (PAS). Since ALPI does not eliminate pupillary block, LPI is still required once IOP is controlled and the cornea has cleared sufficiently. All cases of angle closure originating at any anatomic level (iris-anterior chamber; ciliary body, lens, or posterior to the lens) must be presumed to have some element of pupillary block and if this is not eliminated by iridotomy, continued aqueous secretion into the posterior chamber can undo the effect of ALPI and angle closure can recur.

All published series have reported virtually 100% success at eliminating acute angle closure. In a prospective study of 10 eyes with medically unbreakable attacks lasting 2 to 5 days, mean prelaser IOP was 54.9 mmHg and 2 to 4 hours post-laser was 18.9 mmHg [13]. Even when extensive PAS are present, the IOP is usually normalized within an hour or two. The effect lasts sufficiently long for the cornea and anterior chamber to clear so that iridotomy can be performed, usually by 2 days.

ALPI may also be used as initial therapy in eyes with AAC, either with or without preliminary medical treatment [1, 13–19]. Immediate ALPI for acute attacks after initial treatment with 4% pilocarpine and 0.5% timolol has been reported successful when given over both 180 degrees [17] and 360 degrees of the peripheral iris [15]. This implies that any opacification obstructing laser access to part of the peripheral iris, e.g., by pterygium, still provides enough access for the successful performance of ALPI. Immediate diode laser peripheral iridoplasty in conjunction with topical medications is also successful [20]. The diode laser may be more effective at tissue penetration in the presence of a hazy cornea [21]. Pattern scanning laser (PASCAL) has also been reported successful in treating plateau iris syndrome [22].

ALPI is a safe and effective alternative to glaucoma medications as an initial treatment of AAC [16, 22]. A randomized trial comparing ALPI and medications was performed in consecutive patients diagnosed with AAC with a presenting IOP >40 mmHg, who were not amenable to immediate LPI [16] After initial treatment of 4% pilocarpine and 0.5% timolol in the AAC eye, the patients were randomized to immediate ALPI (33 eyes of 32 patients) or intravenous acetazolamide followed by oral acetazolamide (40 eyes of 32 patients), until IOP normalized. If the presenting IOP was >60 mmHg, the latter group also received intravenous mannitol. In the ALPI-treated group, the mean IOP was reduced from 60.8 ± 11.6 mmHg at presentation to 20.6 ± 10.1 mmHg 1 hour after the procedure. The ALPI-treated group had significantly lower IOP than the medically treated group at 15 minutes, 30 minutes, and 1 hour after initiation of treatment (Fig. 6.2). The reduction in IOP was not affected by the duration of the attack. No significant differences between the two groups in mean IOP, requirement for glaucoma medications, or the extent of PAS was identified upon longer follow-up (mean 15.7 months) [23]. Sng et al. found that immediate ALPI for APAC produced a greater increase in angle width compared to medical therapy [24].

It should be stressed that since ALPI does not eliminate pupillary block, a laser peripheral iridotomy is still required in AAC eyes once IOP is controlled and the cornea has cleared sufficiently.

6.3.1.2 Chronic Angle Closure

Eyes with chronic angle closure (CAC) and a combination of PAS and appositional closure can respond to ALPI with the opening of the appositionally closed portions of the angle. Of 11 eyes with IOP >20 mmHg despite maximal medical therapy, all responded with initial lowering of IOP and 7 remained controlled at 6 months, while 4 required trabeculectomy [25]. In a study comparing the long-term clinical course in eyes with optic nerve head and visual field damage in patients in New York and Singapore, 31.3% of the New York eyes went on to filtering surgery compared to 53.0% of the Singapore eyes [26]. Seven eyes in the New York group underwent

Fig. 6.2 Randomized controlled trial comparing ALPI against conventional systemic IOP-lowering medications as first-line treatment of AAC— Profiles of mean IOP before and at various time points after commencement of treatment in the two treatment groups [15]

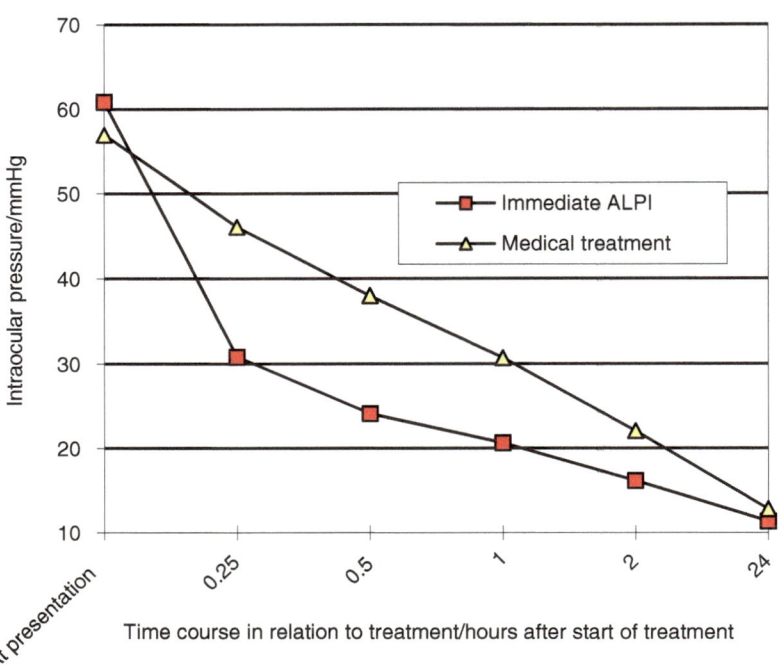

ALPI, after which IOPs were controlled and surgery was not required, while ALPI was not performed in the Singapore patients.

Chen et al. looked at patients treated with LPI with or without ALPI followed >12 months and found IOP fluctuations greatest in patients with PACG versus PAC and correlated with baseline IOP [27]. Cho et al. reported greater angle widening after both LPI and ALPI compared to LPI alone [28]. In a randomized series, Bourne et al. examined 22 patients with gonioscopically occludable angles after LPI. ALPI widened all angle parameters and diurnal IOP measurements were significantly lowered in eyes receiving ALPI compared to those receiving LPI only [29]. Similarly, Ramakrishnan et al. treated 24 eyes with PAC or plateau iris syndrome unresponsive to LPI [30]. ALPI improved angle parameters, lowered mean IOP, and reduced the number of anti-glaucoma medications required.

ALPI can be successful at lowering IOP even when extensive PAS are present, and if this is the case, goniosynechialysis (GSL) may be performed. GSL is a surgical procedure stripping PAS from the angle wall intending to restore

aqueous access to the trabecular meshwork. GSL is thought to be useful only if the PAS have been present for less than 1 year [27]. Literature has shown promising results in both phakic and pseudophakic eyes [20, 28–35]. It is effective as a stand-alone procedure or in conjunction with other surgical procedures, such as cataract extraction [20, 28, 29, 36]. In eyes having had AAC with PAS, combined cataract extraction and GSL was more effective than GSL alone [37]. It is also effective when only the inferior 180 degrees of PAS are re-opened [20, 29]. In one study, 13 patients with IOP >21 mmHg (30.2 ± 8.1) without medications and PAS >180° (301.8 ± 66.5) after phacoemulsification with posterior chamber intraocular lens implantation underwent GSL. At the final follow-up (27.1 ± 17.8 months) after GSL, IOP was <21 mmHg in 10 eyes (13.6 ± 2.3 mmHg) without and in 3 with medications. The mean extent of PAS in the patients with controlled IOP without medications was reduced to 78.6 ± 14.6 degrees. It was concluded that GSL further improves the success by eliminating the need for glaucoma medications and that performing the two procedures simultaneously should be more advantageous than performing them separately [37]. When GSL is performed as a standalone procedure, there is a tendency for the iris to become reapposed to the trabecular meshwork and cause the GSL to fail [37]. Peripheral iridoplasty can be performed postoperatively to further flatten the peripheral iris and prevent synechial reattachment [20, 28, 29, 36]. More recently, especially with long-standing PAS, we have been attempting to perform lens extraction, GSL, and angle procedure, such as a Kahook blade to open the meshwork. When PAS form, the superficial iris tends to grow into the intertrabecular spaces, blocking them, and clearing out the meshwork may allow GSL to be effective when PAS have been present for a longer time.

6.3.2 Secondary Angle Closure Glaucomas

6.3.2.1 Plateau Iris Syndrome

An anteriorly positioned or large ciliary body can result in close proximity between the iris root and the trabecular meshwork, creating a configuration known as plateau iris [38–41]. On gonioscopy, the iris root angulates forward and then centrally. In plateau iris syndrome [42], the angle remains appositionally closed or occludable despite LPI. Before iridotomy, the anterior chamber is usually of medium depth while the iris surface is mildly convex. If pupillary block is either not a component mechanism of the angle closure or that it has been eliminated by iridotomy, physical blockage of the angle can be eliminated by ALPI, which compresses the iris root and creates a space where there was none before (Fig. 6.1).

Long-term success of ALPI has been reported in eyes with plateau iris syndrome [43]. After only one treatment, the angle in 20 eyes out of 23 eyes (87.0%) remained open throughout follow-up (mean follow-up of 79 months) [43]. In the remaining three eyes, gradual re-closure of the angle was noted years later, but they were readily re-opened and maintained open by a single repeat treatment. In all patients, no filtration surgery was necessary during follow-up.

A combined laser technique, with ALPI and sequential LPI in one sitting, has been proposed as initial treatment for eyes with plateau iris syndrome [44]. However, we do not advocate this technique, as one cannot always differentiate plateau iris configuration from plateau iris syndrome; thus the latter cannot be diagnosed until after LPI has been performed, and only then if pilocarpine is not used prior to the LPI, so that the angle structures are not affected by the presence of pilocarpine, which can narrow the angle. ALPI has also been shown to be effective in opening up appositionally closed segments of the drainage angle in plateau-like iris configuration resulting from iridociliary cysts [45, 46]. In some cases, ALPI may fail [47] or recur [48]. It is important to note that if cysts are left unopened, they may continue to enlarge. Our procedure is to perform iridotomies into larger cysts to allow them to drain.

When ALPI is used to open appositionally closed segments of the angle in the presence of a patent iridotomy, a shorter duration of angle closure prior to treatment may be associated with a higher success rate [47].

6.3.3 Lens-Related Angle Closure Glaucoma (Phacomorphic Glaucoma)

Angle closure caused by an enlarged lens or pressure posterior to the lens (malignant glaucoma, aqueous misdirection, ciliary block) is not often responsive to iridotomy, although a component of pupillary block may be present and should be eliminated by iridotomy. These include angle closure secondary to ciliary block, intumescent lens, anterior lens subluxation, or anterior lens displacement secondary to ciliary body edema from acquired immunodeficiency syndrome or ophthalmic procedures such as panretinal photocoagulation or scleral buckling procedures. These situations in which the angle remains appositionally closed after LPI, the apposition can often be partially or entirely eliminated by iridoplasty [3, 4, 47, 49]. After angle opening and IOP reduction, cycloplegics may be given cautiously to ascertain the mechanism of the angle closure. Further definitive surgical intervention such as lens surgery may be necessary after ALPI. However, in secondary malignant glaucoma induced by conditions such as supraciliary effusion after panretinal photocoagulation, the edema usually resolves after a few weeks and observation usually suffices after ALPI and LPI have been performed.

ALPI is also effective as an initial treatment to break acute phacomorphic angle closure attacks [1, 50–52]. In a prospective case series, 10 consecutive patients with acute phacomorphic angle closure received topical atropine (1%), timolol (0.5%), and immediate ALPI as initial treatment [50]. After ALPI, the mean IOP was reduced from 56.1 ± 12.5 mmHg to 37.6 ± 7.5 mmHg at 30 minutes, 25.5 ± 8.7 mmHg at 120 minutes, and 13.6 ± 4.2 mmHg at 1 day. All 10 patients had uncomplicated cataract extraction soon after ALPI. No complications from the laser procedure were encountered.

In a more recent randomized controlled trial, 10 consecutive patients with acute phacomorphic angle closure were randomized to receive either ALPI or systemic carbonic anhydrase inhibitor as initial treatment [52]. In this study, the ALPI-treated group took significantly less time to achieve an IOP of less than 25 mmHg (18.8 ± 7.5 minutes versus 115.0 ± 97.0 minutes, $P = 0.001$, F test), and had a significantly greater IOP reduction within 30 minutes ($69.8\% \pm 7.7\%$ versus $40.9\% \pm 23.9\%$, $p = 0.03$, t-test). The authors concluded that ALPI may offer greater safety, consistency, and efficacy than systemic IOP-lowering medications as initial treatment for acute phacomorphic angle closure.

In acute phacomorphic angle closure, the eye is very often severely inflamed, as these patients have usually been referred after being treated unsuccessfully for a few days. Breaking the attack with ALPI may allow a week or more for the inflammation and folds in Descemet's to clear, permitting cataract extraction under conditions much closer to ideal. Any element of pupillary block is treated with LPI as soon as possible (usually within 2 to 3 days) after breaking the attack.

6.3.4 Nanophthalmos

These patients are anatomically predisposed to angle closure due to anterior chamber crowding. Choroidal effusions and ciliary block may occur following intraocular surgical procedures. If appositional closure persists after LPI, ALPI is indicated. Prophylactic iridotomy is not without risk. Bilateral non-rhegmatogenous retinal detachments have been described following LPI in these patients [53] and maybe attributable to the worsening of preexisting retinal or choroidal disease [54].

6.3.5 Other Uses

ALPI has been reported useful in dealing with various clinical situations, including improving visual function following multifocal intraocular lens implantation [55], treatment of optic obstruction in eyes with the Boston keratoprosthesis [56], in UGH syndrome [57], as an adjunct to goniosynechialysis, in angle closure associated with a cobblestone iris configuration [58–63], and for acute angle closure secondary to treatment with topiramate [64, 65].

6.4 Contraindications

6.4.1 Severe and Extensive Corneal Edema or Opacification

In AAC, a moderate degree of corneal edema is not a contraindication to ALPI. If necessary, glycerine may help clear the cornea temporarily to facilitate performing the procedure. When ALPI is used in aborting AAC attack, partial treatment to only 180° of the peripheral iris may be sufficient as an initial treatment, and so obstruction to optical access to part of the peripheral iris, e.g., by pterygium, need not be a contraindication to ALPI [17].

6.4.2   Flat Anterior Chamber

Corneal endothelial burns can occur when heat is generated at the site of laser burn which in turn heats up the aqueous humor refluxing toward the corneal endothelium. If the iris is apposed to the cornea, any attempt at photocoagulation will result in direct damage to the corneal endothelium. If the anterior chamber is very shallow, laser applications should be timed enough apart to allow the dissipation of heat generated.

6.4.3   Synechial Angle Closure

ALPI is successful in relieving appositional closure, but not synechial closure secondary to PAS formation in eyes with uveitis, neovascular glaucoma, or the iridocorneal-endothelial (ICE) syndrome. Although ALPI has been reported to break PAS [66], we have not been able to accomplish this.

Table 6.1 summarizes the indications and contraindications for ALPI.

Table 6.1 The indications and contraindications for ALPI

Indications for ALPI	Contraindications for ALPI
Acute angle closure	Severe and extensive
Chronic angle closure	corneal edema or opacity
Plateau iris syndrome	Flat anterior chamber
Angle closure due to	Synechial angle closure
position or size of the lens	
Malignant glaucoma	
Nanophthalmos	

6.5   Techniques of ALPI

6.5.1   Pretreatment Measures

The eye is pretreated with topical brimonidine to blunt a post-laser IOP spike and miotic agent to constrict the pupil using one drop of 4% pilocarpine or, if the patient has never had pilocarpine previously, two drops of 2% administered 5 minutes apart. In AAC eyes, moderate degree of corneal edema is not contraindicated to this procedure. If necessary, glycerin can be applied to help clear the cornea temporarily to improve optical access.

6.5.2   Laser Parameters

The argon laser is set to produce contraction burns (500 μm spot size, 0.5 to 0.7 second duration, and, initially 240 mW power). The beam is then aimed at the most peripheral portion of the iris possible (Fig. 6.3) using the Abraham iridotomy contact lens. One of the most common errors resulting in failure of the procedure is wrongful spot placement in the mid-periphery of the iris rather than the extreme periphery. A thin crescent of the aiming beam is allowed to overlap the sclera at the limbus. The patient may be directed to look toward the direction of the beam to achieve more peripheral spot placement. In the lower 240 degrees of angle, the peripheral iris insertion into the angle wall can often be seen directly through the button on the lens, facilitating peripheral aiming beam placement.

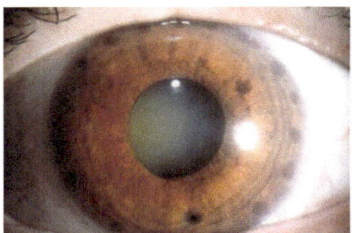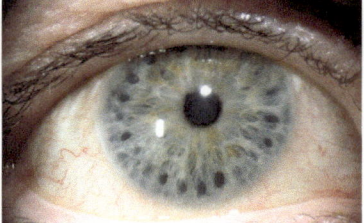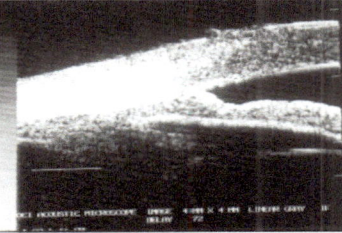

Fig. 6.3 Left: Slit-lamp photograph of an eye with plateau iris syndrome after ALPI. The dark, round laser marks can be clearly seen on the peripheral iris. Center: ALPI being placed too centrally, and thus ineffective. Right: UBM showing APLI being placed too centrally, and the angle remains closed

It is important to ensure that the foot pedal or trigger to be pressed and maintained for the entire duration of the burn, unless there is bubble formation or pigment release. The contraction effect is immediate and usually accompanied by noticeable deepening of the peripheral anterior chamber at the site of the burn. The patient should be warned about mild discomfort upon laser application to induce adequate iris contraction. A lack of visible contraction or deepening of the peripheral anterior chamber at any site is suggestive of inadequate power or PAS. The power should therefore be increased initially to see if contraction can be achieved, particularly if the patient does not feel the burn. To the contrary, power should be reduced if bubble formation occurs or if the pigment is released into the anterior chamber. Histopathologic examination suggests that the short-term effect is related to heat shrinkage of collagen and the long-term effect to be secondary to the contraction of a fibroblastic membrane in the region of the laser application [67].

Lighter irides generally require more power than darker ones upon ALPI. Surgeon should adjust the power as necessary to obtain visible stromal contraction. Occasionally, in light gray irides, a smaller spot size (such as 200 µm) may be more effective in achieving significant stromal contraction. However, the use of a smaller spot size requires more burns to achieve 360° contraction and, particularly with high power settings, may result in stromal destruction and pigment release.

Treatment consists of placing approximately 20–24 spots over 360°, leaving 2 spot-diameters between each spot and avoiding large visible radial vessels if possible. Although rare, iris necrosis may occur if too many spots are placed in close proximity. If the initial treatment is insufficient, more spots may be given at a later sitting. The presence of an arcus senilis should be ignored while performing ALPI. An extremely shallow anterior chamber and corneal edema, which are relative contraindications to laser iridotomy, do not preclude ALPI.

Other laser settings published for ALPI, most commonly 200 µm, 0.1 or 0.2 second duration and 200–800 mW power, often provide insuffi-

cient iris contraction and result in bubble formation or pigment liberation into the anterior chamber. When used through the angled mirror of a gonioscopy lens, they are more likely to result in stromal destruction or inadvertent damage to the trabecular meshwork. The laser beam strikes the iris tangentially and results in a more diffused burn with less peripheral stromal contraction.

Two additional situations should be noted. First, repeated ALPI is sometimes needed because of recurrence of appositional closure at some point after the angle has been initially opened, it is then possible to place the contraction burns further peripherally than had been initially possible. The reason for this is evident if one conceptualizes the geometry of the peripheral iris. When the angle is closed, burns have to be placed inside the point of apposition in order to pull open the angle and expose iris stroma further peripherally. If necessary, this area can be treated on a subsequent occasion.

Secondly, a few angles have a very sharply defined plateau, which on indentation forms almost a right angle and requires firm pressure to indent open. This type of plateau iris often does not completely react to contraction burns placed with the Abraham lens but require burns placed through one of the angled mirrors with magnification buttons of the Ritch lens or Goldmann 3-mirror lens directly into the peripheral angle. A 200 µm spot size should be used in this circumstance.

In some cases, we can perform ALPI without using pilocarpine. With the technician shining a bright light, such as that from a scleral fiberoptic transilluminator, into the pupil of the fellow eye, and, with the consensual light reflex in effect in the eye to be lasered, ALPI is performed directly into the angle with the Ritch lens using 0.5–0.7 second, 200 microns spot size, and, initially, 240 mW power. The advantage of this method is that the laser outcomes and angle status can be immediately visualized with settings adjusted throughout the procedure to open the angle.

Apart from argon laser, the use of diode laser [19] and double-frequency Nd:YAG laser [68, 69] in laser peripheral iridoplasty to treat appositional angle closure have also been described.

6.5.3 Postoperative Treatment

Immediately after the procedure, the patient is given a drop of topical steroid and apraclonidine or brimonidine. Gonioscopy should be performed to assess the effect of the procedure immediately if pilocarpine has not been used. If it has, it is better to evaluate the success of the procedure at a subsequent visit. Patients are treated with topical steroids 4 to 6 times daily for 3 to 5 days. Intraocular pressure is monitored postoperatively as after any other anterior segment laser procedure and patients treated as necessary if a post-laser IOP rise occurs.

6.6 Complications of ALPI and Management

A mild postoperative iritis is common and responds to topical steroid treatment, seldom lasting more than a few days. The patient may experience transient ocular irritation.

As iridoplasty is often performed on patients with extremely shallow peripheral anterior chambers, diffuse corneal endothelial burns can sometimes occur. As opposed to the dense white, sharply delineated burns seen during laser iridotomy, endothelial burns noted during ALPI are larger and much less opaque. If endothelial burns are identified early in the procedure, they may be minimized by placing an initial contraction burn more centrally before placing the peripheral burn (kriss-kross iridoplasty). This first burn will deepen the anterior chamber peripheral to it, allowing the placement of the more peripheral burn with less adverse consequences. In virtually all cases, the endothelial burns disappear within several days and have not proven to be a major complication [16]. Among thousands of ALPI performed, we have only seen one case of corneal decompensation following ALPI in a patient with preexisting Fuchs' dystrophy.

Hemorrhage seldomly occurs because of the lower power used to produce contraction burns as opposed to destructive ones [16]. Nevertheless, a transient rise in IOP can happen as with other anterior segment laser procedures. Lenticular opacification has not been reported.

Pigmented burn marks may develop at the sites of laser applications in some eyes treated with ALPI and are generally of no serious consequence [18]. Iris atrophy may rarely develop [18], and this can be avoided by using the lowest laser power to achieve stromal contraction, and also by leaving adequate untreated spaces between two laser application sites, and not allowing the laser marks to become confluent. Upon rapid IOP reduction by ALPI in acute primary angle closure, decompression retinopathy can rarely occur [23, 70].

Some patients have developed slight to moderately dilated pupils post-laser (Urrets-Zavalia syndrome), enough to cause photophobia and/or anxiety over the appearance or to threaten a recurrence of angle closure. Pilocarpine 2% may be administered to reduce the pupil size. This does not necessarily work in all cases, but in our experience, the pupil size has normalized in all the cases, although this has occasionally taken months [71]. If the fellow eye is felt to need ALPI and the patient is willing, we will proceed. We do not know the mechanism underlying this complication, although a similar event has been reported following peripheral retinal laser treatment [72].

Asymmetry of eyes with narrow angles occurs because of differences in iris insertion position on the ciliary body face and from asymmetry of the ciliary body position [73]. Plateau iris configuration and even iridociliary apposition may persist after cataract extraction [74]. Angle closure may rarely recur in these eyes [75]

Although ALPI is highly successful long term in eyes with plateau iris, patients need to be followed closely for recurrence of appositional closure, and if this develops, may require retreatment. Patients should be observed gonioscopically at regular intervals and further treatment given if necessary. This is most common in a patient in whom the mechanism of the glaucoma is lens-related or as the lens enlarges over time. Retreatment is only occasionally needed in patients with plateau iris [43], while those with intumescent lenses usually undergo cataract extraction.

6.7   Conclusions

ALPI is a safe and simple out-patient laser procedure that effectively opens appositionally closed portions of the drainage angle. Since it does not eliminate pupillary block, laser peripheral iridotomy is still indicated if pupillary block is present.

ALPI has taken on new indications in recent years. It is now a viable alternative first-line treatment for AAC, in place of systemic IOP-lowering medications. It reduces IOP more rapidly than medications. Ongoing studies will tell whether ALPI can also reduce the rate of conversion to CACG after AAC. ALPI may also have a role in the treatment of acute phacomorphic angle closure in the future. It is essential to keep in mind that lower power, longer duration, and larger spot sizes (contraction burns) are the most effective in achieving success with this procedure.

References

1. Ritch R. Argon laser treatment for medically unresponsive attacks of angle-closure glaucoma. Am J Ophthalmic. 1982;94:197–204.
2. Ritch R. Techniques of argon laser iridectomy and iridoplasty. Palo Alto: Coherent Medical Press; 1983.
3. York K, Ritch R, Szmyd LJ. Argon laser peripheral iridoplasty: indications, techniques and results. Invest Ophthalmol Vis Sci. 1984;25(Suppl):94.
4. Ritch R, Solomon IS. Glaucoma surgery. In: L'Esperance FA, editor. Ophthalmic lasers. 3rd ed. St. Louis: CV Mosby Co; 1989.
5. Ritch R. Argon laser peripheral iridoplasty: an overview. J Glaucoma. 1992;1:206–13.
6. Ritch R, Liebmann JM, Tello C. A construct for understanding angle-closure glaucoma: the role of ultrasound biomicroscopy. Ophthalmol Clin N Amer. 1995;8:281–93.
7. Krasnov MM. Q-switched laser iridectomy and Q-switched laser goniopuncture. Adv Ophthalmol. 1977;34:192–6.
8. Kimbrough RL, Trempe CS, Brockhurst RJ, Simmons RJ. Angle-closure glaucoma in nanophthalmos. Am J Ophthalmol. 1979;88:572–9.
9. Ritch R, Tham CCY, Lam DSC. Argon laser peripheral iridoplasty – update 2007. Surv Ophthalmol. 2007;52:279–88.
10. Matai A, Consul S. Argon laser iridoplasty. Indian J Ophthalmol. 1987;35:290–2.
11. Malis V. Importance of laser peripheral iridoplasty in the treatment of acute closed-angle glaucoma. Ceska a Slovenska Oftalmolgie. 2001;57:22–6.
12. Lim AS, Tan A, Chew P, et al. Laser iridoplasty in the treatment of severe acute angle closure glaucoma. Int Ophthalmol. 1993;17:33–6.
13. Chew P, Chee C, Lim A. Laser treatment of severe acute angle-closure glaucoma in dark Asian irides: the role of iridoplasty. Lasers Light Ophthalmol. 1991;4:41–2.
14. Agarwal HC, Kumar R, Kalra VK, Sood NN. Argon laser iridoplasty: a primary mode of therapy in primary angle-closure glaucoma. Indian J Ophthalmol. 1991;39:87–90.
15. Lam DS, Lai JS, Tham CC. Immediate argon laser peripheral iridoplasty as treatment for acute attack of primary angle-closure glaucoma. A preliminary study. Ophthalmology. 1998;105:2231–6.
16. Lam DS, Lai JS, Tham CC, et al. Argon laser peripheral iridoplasty versus conventional systemic medical therapy as the first line treatment of acute angle closure: a prospective randomized controlled trial. Ophthalmology. 2002;109:1591–6.
17. Lai JS, Tham CC, Lam DS. Limited argon laser peripheral iridoplasty as immediate treatment for an acute attack of angle-closure glaucoma: a preliminary study. Eye. 1999;13:26–30.
18. Lai JS, Tham CC, Chua JK, et al. Laser peripheral iridoplasty as initial treatment of acute attack of primary angle-closure: a long-term follow-up study. J Glaucoma. 2002;11:484–7.
19. Tham CC, Lai JS, Lam DS. Immediate ALPI for acute attack of angle-closure glaucoma (addendum to previous report). Ophthalmology. 1999;106:1042–3.
20. Lai JS, Tham CC, Chua JK, Lam DS. Immediate diode laser peripheral iridoplasty as treatment of acute attack of primary angle-closure glaucoma. A preliminary study. J Glaucoma. 2001;10:89–94.
21. Chew PT, Wong JS, Chee CK, Tock EP. Corneal transmissibility of diode versus argon lasers and their photothermal effects on the cornea and iris. Clin Exp Ophthalmol. 2000;28:53–7.
22. Midha N, Hoskens K, Mansouri K. Pattern scanning laser (PASCAL) for peripheral iridoplasty in eyes with plateau iris syndrome: a novel application. J Glaucoma. 2018 Jul;27(7):e124–7.
23. Lai JS, Tham CC, Chua JK, et al. To compare argon laser peripheral iridoplasty (ALPI) against systemic medications in treatment of acute primary angle-closure: mid-term results. Eye. 2006 Mar;20(3):309–14.
24. Sng CC, Aquino MC, Liao J, et al. Anterior segment morphology after acute primary angle closure treatment: a randomised study comparing iridoplasty and medical therapy. Br J Ophthalmol. 2016;100:542–8.
25. Chew PT, Yeo LM. Argon laser iridoplasty in chronic angle-closure glaucoma. Int Ophthalmol. 1995;19:67–70.
26. Rosman M, Aung T, Ang LP, et al. Chronic angle-closure with glaucomatous damage: long-term clinical course in a north American population and com-

parison with an Asian population. Ophthalmology. 2002;109:2227–31.

27. Chen YY, Sun LP, Thomas R, et al. Long-term intraocular pressure fluctuation of primary angle closure disease following laser peripheral iridotomy/iridoplasty. Chin Med J. 2011;124(19):3066–9.

28. Cho HK, Kee C, Yang H, et al. Comparison of circumferential peripheral angle closure using iridotrabecular contact index after laser iridotomy versus combined laser iridotomy and iridoplasty. Acta Ophthalmol. 2017;95(7):e539–47.

29. Bourne RR, Zhekov I, Pardhan S. Temporal ocular coherence tomography-measured changes in anterior chamber angle and diurnal intraocular pressure after laser iridoplasty: IMPACT study. Br J Ophthalmol. 2017;101:886–91.

30. Ramakrishnan R, Mitra A, Abdul Kader M, Das S. To study the efficacy of laser peripheral iridoplasty in the treatment of eyes with primary angle closure and plateau iris syndrome, unresponsive to laser peripheral iridotomy, using anterior-segment OCT as a tool. J Glaucoma. 2016 May;25(5):440–6.

31. Campbell DG, Vela A. Modern goniosynechialysis for the treatment of synechial angle-closure glaucoma. Ophthalmology. 1984;91:1052–60.

32. Kanamori A, Nakamura M, Matsui N, et al. Goniosynechialysis with lens aspiration and posterior intraocular lens implantation for glaucoma in spherophakia. J Cataract Refract Surg. 2004;30:513–6.

33. Lai JS, Tham CC, Chua JK, Lam DS. Efficacy and safety of inferior 180° goniosynechialysis followed by diode laser peripheral iridoplasty in the treatment of chronic angle-closure glaucoma. J Glaucoma. 2000;9:388–91.

34. Nagata M, Nezu N. Goniosynechialysis as a new treatment for chronic angle-closure glaucoma. Jpn J Clin Ophthalmol. 1985;39:707–10.

35. Ando H, Kitagawa K, Ogino N. Results of goniosynechialysis for synechial angle-closure glaucoma after pupillary block. Folia Ophthalmol Jpn. 1990;41:883–6.

36. Tanihara H, Nishiwaki K, Nagata M. Surgical results and complications of goniosynechialysis. Graefes Arch Clin Exp Ophthalmol. 1992;230:309–13.

37. Teekhasaenee C, Ritch R. Combined phacoemulsification and goniosynechialysis for uncontrolled chronic angle-closure glaucoma after acute angle-closure glaucoma. Ophthalmology. 1999;106:669–75.

38. Tornquist R. Angle-closure glaucoma in an eye with a plateau type of iris. Acta Ophthalmol. 1958;36:419–23.

39. Wand M, Pavlin CJ, Foster FS. Plateau iris syndrome: ultrasound biomicroscopic and histological study. Ophthalmic Surg. 1993;24:129–31.

40. Ritch R. Plateau iris is caused by abnormally positioned ciliary processes. J Glaucoma. 1992;1:23–6.

41. Pavlin CJ, Ritch R, Foster FS. Ultrasound biomicroscopy in plateau iris syndrome. Am J Ophthalmol. 1992;113:390–5.

42. Lowe RF, Ritch R. Angle-closure glaucoma: clinical types. In: Ritch R, Shields MB, Krupin T, editors. The Glaucomas. St. Louis: CV Mosby Co; 1989. p. 839–53.

43. Ritch R, Tham CC, Lam DS. Long-term success of argon laser peripheral iridoplasty in the management of plateau iris syndrome. Ophthalmology. 2004;111:104–8.

44. Peng D, Zhang X, Yu K. Argon laser peripheral iridoplasty and laser iridectomy for plateau iris glaucoma. Chung Hua Yen Ko Tsa Chih. 1997;33:165–8. Chinese

45. Crowston JG, Medeiros FA, Mosaed S, Weinreb RN. Argon laser iridoplasty in the treatment of plateau-like iris configuration as result of numerous ciliary body cysts. Am J Ophthalmol. 2005;139:381–3.

46. Suriano MM. Plateau iris secondary to iridociliary cysts. Arch Soc Esp Oftalmol. 2015;90(11):542–5. Epub Apr 22

47. Ang GS, Bochmann F, Azuara-Blanco A. Argon laser peripheral iridoplasty for plateau iris associated with iridociliary cysts: a case report. Cases J. 2008;1(1):368.

48. Ispa-Callἀn MC, Lara-Medina J, Zarco-Tejada JM, et al. Argon laser iridoplasty as treatment of plateau-like iris configuration secondary to multiple ciliary body cysts: long-term follow-up by ultrasound biomicroscopy. Arch Soc Esp Oftalmol. 2009;84(11):569–72.

49. Burton TC, Folk JC. Laser iris retraction for angle-closure glaucoma after retinal detachment surgery. Ophthalmology. 1988;95:742–8.

50. Tham CC, Lai JS, Poon AS, et al. Immediate argon laser peripheral iridoplasty (ALPI) as initial treatment for acute phacomorphic angle-closure (phacomorphic glaucoma) before cataract extraction: a preliminary study. Eye (Lond). 2005;19:778–83.

51. Yip PP, Leung WY, Hon CY, Ho CK. Argon laser peripheral iridoplasty in the management of phacomorphic glaucoma. Ophthalmic Surg Lasers Imaging. 2005;36:286–91.

52. Lee JW, Lai JS, Yick DW, Yuen CY. Argon laser peripheral iridoplasty versus systemic intraocular pressure-lowering medications as immediate management for acute phacomorphic angle closure. Clin Ophthalmol. 2013;7:63–9. https://doi.org/10.2147/OPTH.S39503. Epub 2013 Jan 9

53. Karjalainen K, Laatikainen L, Raitta C. Bilateral nonrhegmatogenous retinal detachment following neodymium-YAG laser iridotomies. Arch Ophthalmol. 1986;104:1134.

54. Singh OS, Belcher CD, Simmons RJ. Nanophthalmic eyes and neodymium-YAG laser iridectomies. Arch Ophthalmol. 1987;105:455–6.

55. Solomon R, Barsam A, Voldman A, et al. Argon laser iridoplasty to improve visual function following multifocal intraocular lens implantation. J Refract Surg. 2012;28(4):281–3. https://doi.org/10.3928/108159 7X-20120209-01. Epub 2012 Feb 15

56. Kang JJ, Allemann N, Cortina MS, et al. Argon laser iridoplasty for optic obstruction of Boston keratoprosthesis. Arch Ophthalmol. 2012;130(8):1051–4.

57. Walland MJ. Uveitis-glaucoma-hyphaema (UGH) syndrome treated with local laser iridoplasty. Clin Exp Ophthalmol. 2017 Aug;45(6):647–8.

58. Kameda T, Inoue T, Inatani M, et al. Long-term efficacy of goniosynechialysis combined with phacoemulsification for primary angle closure. Graefes Arch Clin Exp Ophthalmol 251(3):825-830. 2012 Jun 29. Epub ahead of print.

59. Kanamori A, Nakamura M, Matsui N, et al. Goniosynechialysis with lens aspiration and posterior intraocular lens implantation for glaucoma in spherophakia. J Cataract Refract Surg. 2004;30:513–6.

60. Lai JS, Tham CC, Chua JK, Lam DS. Efficacy and safety of inferior 180° goniosynechialysis followed by diode laser peripheral iridoplasty in the treatment of chronic angle-closure glaucoma. J Glaucoma. 2000;9:388–91.

61. Lai JS, Tham CC, Lam DS. The efficacy and safety of combined phacoemulsification, intraocular lens implantation, and limited goniosynechialysis, followed by diode laser peripheral iridoplasty, as the treatment of cataract and chronic angle-closure glaucoma. J Glaucoma. 2001;10:309–15.

62. Tanihara H, Nagata M. Argon-laser gonioplasty following goniosynechialysis. Graefes Arch Clin Exp Ophthalmol. 1991;229:505–7.

63. Prata TS, Biteli LG, Dorairaj S. Angle closure associated with a cobblestone iris configuration: clinical and imaging description. J Glaucoma. 2013 Dec;22(9):e36–7. https://doi.org/10.1097/01.ijg.0000435777.99193.08.

64. Sbeity Z, Gvozdyuk N, Amde W, et al. Argon laser peripheral iridoplasty for topiramate-induced bilateral acute angle closure. J Glaucoma. 2009;18:269–71.

65. Zalta AH, Smith RT. Peripheral iridoplasty efficacy in refractory topiramate-associated bilateral acute angle-closure glaucoma. Arch Ophthalmol. 2008;126:1603–5.

66. Wand M. Argon laser gonioplasty for synechial angle closure. Arch Ophthalmol. 1992;110:353–7.

67. Sassani JW, Ritch R, McCormick S, et al. Histopathology of argon laser peripheral iridoplasty. Ophthalmic Surg. 1993;24:740–5.

68. Zou J, Zhang F, Zhang L, Wang L, Huang H. A clinical study on laser peripheral iridoplasty for primary angle-closure glaucoma with positive provocative tests after iridectomy. Zhonghua Yan Ke Za Zhi. 2002;38:708–11.

69. Zhang HC, Yao K. Peripheral iridoplasty with doubled-frequency Nd:YAG laser as treatment for angle-closure glaucoma. Zhejiang Da Xue Xue Bao Yi Xue Ban. 2002;31:388–90.

70. Lai JSM, Lee VYW, Leung DYL, Chung ICF. Decompression retinopathy following laser peripheral iridoplasty for acute primary angle-closure. Eye. 2006;19:1345–7.

71. Espana EM, Ioannidis A, Tello C, Liebmann JM, Foster P, Ritch R. Urrets-Zavalia syndrome as a complication of argon laser peripheral iridoplasty. Br J Ophthalmol. 2007;91:427–9.

72. Lifshitz T, Yassur Y. Accommodative weakness and mydriasis following laser treatment at the peripheral retina. Ophthalmologica. 1988;197:65–8.

73. Dorairaj SK, Ritch R, Tello C, et al. Narrow angles and angle closure: anatomic reasons for earlier closure of the superior portion of the iridocorneal angle. Arch Ophthalmol. 2007;125:734–9.

74. Tran HV, Ritch R, Liebmann JM. Iridociliary apposition in plateau iris syndrome persists after cataract extraction. Am J Ophthalmol. 2003;135:40–4.

75. Choy BN, Chan JC, Chien CP, Lai JS. Recurrent acute angle-closure attack due to plateau iris syndrome after cataract extraction with or without argon laser peripheral iridoplasty: a case report. BMC Ophthalmol. 2016;16:640.

The Role of Selective Laser Trabeculoplasty in Primary Angle Closure Glaucoma

Jimmy Shiu Ming Lai

Abstract

Selective laser trabeculoplasty is proven to be safe and effective in the treatment of primary open-angle glaucoma. It reduces intraocular pressure by 20 to 30% from the baseline. However, the role of SLT in the treatment of primary angle-closure glaucoma remains an area worth exploring. Current data have shown it to be effective in selected cases. Nevertheless, there remain many uncertainties in the intraocular pressure response and long-term treatment outcome when SLT is used in the treatment of primary angle closure glaucoma.

Keywords

Selective laser trabeculoplasty · Primary angle closure glaucoma

Selective laser trabeculoplasty (SLT) is an outpatient procedure that reduces intraocular pressure in patients with ocular hypertension and glaucoma. The Q-switched, frequency-doubled Nd:YAG (532 nm) laser is applied through a special contact lens to the trabecular meshwork where it stimulates a biochemical change that increases the aqueous outflow from the anterior chamber. SLT can lower intraocular pressure by 20–30% from the baseline in about 80% of the treated patients. It therefore has a similar efficacy compared to ocular hypotensive eye drops. The intraocular pressure reduction effect may last for 3–5 years after a single treatment and SLT can be repeated when the therapeutic effect diminishes with time. SLT has been indicated as a safe and efficient treatment for primary open-angle glaucoma. Recent studies have also shown its effectiveness in the treatment of primary angle closure glaucoma (PACG). It is possible to apply SLT to angle closure patients who have at least 90 degrees of visible trabecular meshwork either because of incomplete angle closure or angle reopening after laser peripheral iridotomy, lens/cataract extraction, and/or goniosynechialysis. Despite the potential benefits of SLT in selected cases of PACG, the mechanisms underlying the intraocular pressure reduction in these glaucoma cases are still poorly understood.

Ho CL; et al. in 2009 studied whether SLT could lower intraocular pressure in eyes with primary angle closure after laser peripheral iridotomy [1]. In their study, patients with primary angle closure who had undergone laser peripheral iridotomy and who had an intraocular pressure greater than 21 mm Hg and a gonioscopically visible pigmented trabecular meshwork for at least 90 degrees were enrolled. SLT was applied

J. S. M. Lai (✉)
Department of Ophthalmology, The University of Hong Kong, Hong Kong, China
e-mail: laism@hku.hk

© Springer Nature Singapore Pte Ltd. 2021
C. C. Y. Tham (ed.), *Primary Angle Closure Glaucoma (PACG)*,
https://doi.org/10.1007/978-981-15-8120-5_7

to the open-angle segments. It was found that SLT was safe and effective in reducing the intraocular pressure in patients with primary angle closure glaucoma and a patent iridotomy when there was a sufficient extent of the visible trabecular meshwork.

Ali Aljasim L; et al. in 2016 achieved a success rate of 84.7% in PAC/PACG subjects treated with SLT. They defined success as clinically significant intraocular pressure reduction of 20% or more from the baseline or discontinuation of one or more of glaucoma medications in [2]. The success rate was comparable to that of the primary open-angle glaucoma which was 79.6%. However, an IOP spike occurred in 10% in the PAC/PACG groups which were two times more than that of the primary open-angle glaucoma group.

Raj S; et al. in 2018 also showed SLT to be a safe and cost-effective treatment for reducing intraocular pressure in primary angle closure glaucoma in the presence of a patent laser iridotomy and a visible trabecular meshwork [3]. They also found that a high baseline intraocular pressure positively correlated with the degree of intraocular pressure reduction.

However, despite the favorable short-term outcomes of SLT in the treatment of PACG, Kurysheva NI; et al. in 2016 found that the initial success rate was 87% in the first year dropped to 4% in the sixth year after SLT [4]. The long-term outcome of the initial SLT and the repeat SLT in the treatment of PACG needs further evaluation through large controlled clinical trials.

What are the factors that may lead to a different short-term and long-term outcome of SLT in the treatment of PACG compared to primary open-angle glaucoma? The histopathological changes going on in the trabecular meshwork in PACG may differ from those of primary open-angle glaucoma. One cannot translate the SLT outcomes of primary open-angle glaucoma directly to PACG. Theoretically, the SLT response should be better in PACG eyes with incomplete angle closure than in eyes with angle reopened up angle after laser peripheral iridotomy. This is because the peripheral anterior synechiae (PAS) free trabecular meshwork should have less histopathological changes than trabecular meshwork

that had previous PAS closure. In the treatment of PACG patients with SLT, a variable response is expected. This is because the degree of visible trabecular meshwork that can be treated varies in different individuals. Furthermore, it is technically difficult to identify the trabecular meshwork because of irregular pigment deposits in the angle especially after laser peripheral iridotomy. It is also difficult to quantify the degree of the visible trabecular meshwork. Even if the open area is clearly identified and the trabecular meshwork is clearly visualized, there is still less treatable area than in primary open-angle glaucoma. Furthermore, it is not clear how the degree of pigmentation in the angle affects the outcome of SLT.

Since the pathogenesis of the PACG is caused by a relative anatomical derangement of the anterior segment, the treatment strategy aims at the reconstruction of the anatomical defect as well as intraocular pressure control. With the emergence of evidence, early cataract extraction and clear lens extraction have become more affirmative in the treatment of PACG. The role of SLT in the treatment of PACG seems to be trivial. However, SLT may still have a role in the following situations. In ophthalmic centers with long wait list for cataract surgery, SLT may be a useful tool to control the intraocular pressure while patients are waiting for the surgery. In patients who prefer to preserve their clear lens for reading and in patients who will suffer from severe anisometropia after lens removal, SLT may be considered as an alternative to lens extraction. SLT may also have a supplementary role in PACG by modulation of the unhealthy trabecular meshwork after cataract/lens extraction and/or goniosynechialysis. The cataract extraction and the goniosynechialysis serve to reconstruct the anterior segment anatomical defect while SLT revitalizes the trabecular tissue. In PACG eyes with persistently elevated intraocular pressure after angle opening procedures, SLT may be considered in replacement of medical therapy in medically controlled cases and in medically uncontrolled cases, it may be offered before proceeding to glaucoma surgery.

There are limitations of SLT in the treatment of PACG. If there is total angle occlusion or if the visible angle is less than 90 degrees, SLT cannot or should not be used. And SLT cannot be used to treat acute attack of angle closure. SLT should not be used in PACG eyes in which the angle where the visible trabecular meshwork is located is very narrow. This is because of the risk of corneal damage if a large area of the laser spots is placed on the corneal endothelial tissue [5].

SLT alone cannot open a closed angle. It can only be applied to angle where the trabecular meshwork can be visualized. It cannot replace other angle opening procedures that need to be present to minimize the chance of angle reclosure. Therefore, PACG eyes receiving SLT should have a patent laser peripheral iridotomy and/or pseudophakia. Up to date, there is no reported sight-threatening complications directly related to SLT in the treatment of PACG. Provided that we minimize the post-SLT intraocular pressure spike magnitude and duration with medications, it appears to be a safe treatment option for selected cases of PACG. It offers a minimally invasive intervention in intraocular pressure control in PACG.

References

1. Ho CL, Lai JS, Aquino MV, Rojanapongpun P, Wong HT, Aquino MC, Gerber Y, Belkin M, Barkana Y. Selective laser trabeculoplasty for primary angle closure with persistently elevated intraocular pressure after iridotomy. J Glaucoma. 2009 Sep;18(7):563–6.
2. Ali Aljasim L, Owaidhah O, Edward DP. Selective laser Trabeculoplasty in primary angle-closure Glaucoma after laser peripheral Iridotomy: a case-control study. J Glaucoma. 2016 Mar;25(3):e253–8.
3. Raj S, Tigari B, Faisal TT, Gautam N, Kaushik S, Ichhpujani P, Pandav SS, Ram J. Efficacy of selective laser trabeculoplasty in primary angle closure disease. Eye (Lond). 2018 Nov;32(11):1710–6.
4. Kurysheva NI, Lepeshkina LV, Shatalova EO. Predictors of outcome in selective laser Trabeculoplasty: a long-term observation study in primary angle-closure Glaucoma after laser peripheral Iridotomy compared with primary open-angle Glaucoma. J Glaucoma. 2018 Oct;27(10):880–6.
5. Lee JW, Chan JC, Chang RT, Singh K, Liu CC, Gangwani R, Wong MO, Lai JS. Corneal changes after a single session of selective laser trabeculoplasty for open-angle glaucoma. Eye (Lond). 2014 Jan;28(1):47–52.

Lens Extraction in PACG

8

Noel Ching-Yan Chan and Clement C. Y. Tham

Abstract

With the advancement of technology and the development of phacoemulsification, lens extraction can now be performed through smaller corneal incisions with minimal conjunctival manipulation and intraoperative intraocular pressure fluctuations. For different stages of Primary Angle Closure diseases, phacoemulsification alone or combined with glaucoma procedures are important surgical treatment options in the control of intraocular pressure and disease progression. This chapter will illustrate the algorithm in the choice of surgery in different scenarios with the display of recent evidence. We will also discuss the potential perioperative risk and complications aside from its preventive measures in this group of patients.

Keywords

Lens extraction · Angle closure · Cataract Small pupil · Glaucoma

8.1 Introduction

In newly diagnosed primary angle closure diseases, the management principle is to first re-open all appositionally closed portions of the drainage angle by eliminating the key mechanism(s) of angle closure, with the aim of normalizing intraocular pressure (IOP), and preventing further glaucomatous progression. Traditionally, laser peripheral iridotomy (with or without subsequent laser peripheral iridoplasty) is the mainstay in opening up the drainage angle. In this era when phacoemulsification has become a relatively safe and widely practiced procedure, lens extraction has become one of the initial surgical options as well (Fig. 8.1).

8.2 Lens Extraction in Angle Closure Glaucoma

Besides reversing one important anatomical predisposition to angle closure and lowering IOP, there are other potential benefits of lens extraction in Primary Angle Closure Glaucoma

N. C.-Y. Chan (✉)
Department of Ophthalmology and Visual Sciences, Prince of Wales and Alice Ho Miu Ling Nethersole Hospitals, New Territories East Cluster, Hospital Authority, Hong Kong, China

Department of Ophthalmology and Visual Sciences, The Chinese University of Hong Kong, Hong Kong, China

C. C. Y. Tham
Department of Ophthalmology and Visual Sciences, The Chinese University of Hong Kong, Hong Kong, China

Hong Kong Eye Hospital, Hong Kong, Chinae-mail: clemtham@cuhk.edu.hk

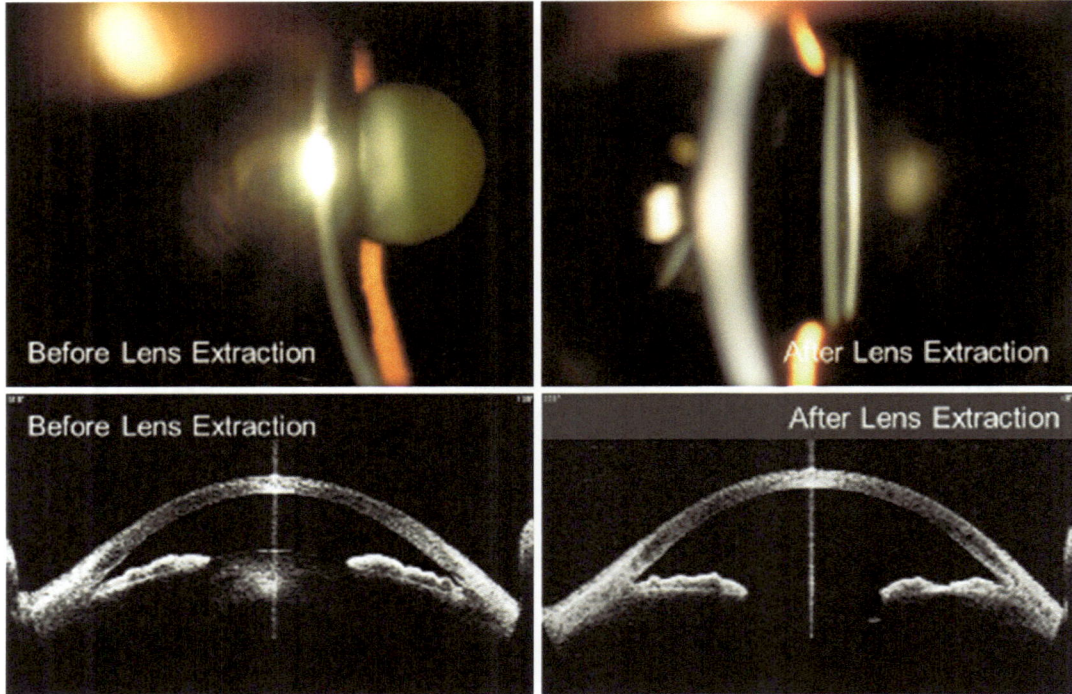

Fig. 8.1 Legend Text: Lens extraction results in deepening of the anterior chamber, opening of appositional angle closure, and reduction of pupillary block

(PACG). It may decrease the need for subsequent glaucoma surgery. It also decreases the risk of complications (including cataract formation) associated with glaucoma surgery. The consensus now is that lens extraction is a beneficial initial or early surgical intervention in most PACG patients [1].

The question of interest comes down to the timing of this intervention and when to consider it in different scenarios requiring surgical intervention:

(a) IOP uncontrolled with drugs + coexisting cataract
(b) IOP controlled with drugs + coexisting cataract
(c) IOP uncontrolled with drugs + no cataract
(d) Newly diagnosed PAC/PACG with high IOP + no cataract
(e) Acute primary angle closure (APAC)

8.3 IOP Uncontrolled with Drugs with Coexisting Cataract

In this scenario, the main surgical options include phacoemulsification alone versus combined phacotrabeculectomy, both of which can reduce IOP in PACG eyes. Trabeculectomy alone has a limited role in this case, because of the known pathogenic role of the lens in PACG, and also because of the relatively higher perioperative risk of complications of performing trabeculectomy in PACG eyes. Furthermore, a significant proportion of patients will soon need cataract extraction after trabeculectomy, and future cataract extraction may result in loss of the functioning filter. Studies have reported that 30–100% of previously functioning blebs will require glaucoma medications to control IOP after subsequent cataract surgery.

A randomized controlled trial revealed that combined surgery resulted in better IOP control than did phacoemulsification alone over a 24-month follow-up period, as suggested by a lower mean IOP and the requirement of 1.2 fewer topical glaucoma medications [2]. However, this difference was not statistically significant at 5 years after surgery [3]. 11.1% and 29.6% of phacoemulsification-alone eyes subsequently required trabeculectomy for IOP control within the 2-year and 5-year period, respectively [2]. There was no significant difference between the two groups in terms of visual acuity or glaucomatous progression at 2 or 5 years follow-up [2, 3]. Yet, combined phaco-trabeculectomy resulted in more postoperative complications, and 25% of these eyes required additional surgical procedures such as laser suture lysis or needling to maintain filtration [2, 3].

Phacoemulsification alone is still a viable first-line surgical option in this setting, but combined phaco-trabeculectomy should be considered in those patients requiring greater IOP reduction or maximum drug reduction. Either approach may be adopted depending on patient factors. For example, phacoemulsification alone may be considered in patients who are more prone to the risk of trabeculectomy complications or in eyes that carry higher surgical risk when subjected to combined surgery (such as eyes with lower endothelial cell count). On the other hand, combined phaco-trabeculectomy would be a good option for patients with poor compliance or accessibility to medications, or those with multiple drug allergies.

8.4   IOP Controlled with Drugs with Coexisting Cataract

The major surgical options are again phacoemulsification alone and combined phaco-trabeculectomy. The efficacy of phacoemulsification alone in widening anterior chamber angles, reducing IOP and drug requirement, has been long studied [4]. In PACG eyes, phacoemulsification alone resulted in greater opening of drainage angle and greater deepening of the anterior chamber than combined phaco-trabeculectomy [5]. A ran-

domized controlled trial has shown that phacoemulsification alone can result in 9.82% IOP reduction and 59.2% drug reduction. Although combined phaco-trabeculectomy resulted in 1.67 mm Hg more IOP reduction and 0.8 fewer topical glaucoma drug requirements, it came with a higher risk of complications [6]. At 5 years after surgery, only 8.6% of the phacoemulsification group required additional glaucoma surgery [3]. Therefore, in this scenario, the benefit of combined phaco-trabeculectomy is probably not sufficient to justify the additional risk of complications and postoperative interventions. Phacoemulsification may be the surgery of choice.

8.5   IOP Uncontrolled with Drugs and with No Cataract

"Clear lens extraction" is the term commonly used to describe the extraction of an optically clear lens when there is no visually significant cataract. The word "clear" emphasizes that the visual acuity is not sufficiently affected by the lens status. However, the pathophysiology of PACG often includes an abnormally thick and anteriorly positioned lens, which results in an exaggerated pupillary block (Fig. 8.1). The lens is thus a crucial component in the pathogenesis of PACG and should be considered pathological in PACG, despite its clarity. Therefore, in this scenario, the surgical options may include trabeculectomy alone or phacoemulsification alone.

For this group of patients, it has been shown that clear lens extraction resulted in a significant reduction in synechial angle closure, and an increase in anterior chamber angle width and anterior chamber depth compared to trabeculectomy alone [7]. A randomized controlled trial has shown that phacoemulsification alone is effective in reducing IOP by 34% and glaucoma drug requirement by 59.5% [8]. Over the first 24 months, trabeculectomy has a similar IOP lowering effect as phacoemulsification alone and can lead to 1.06 fewer glaucoma medications. Eyes receiving trabeculectomy have a higher surgical complication rate of 45.8% as compared to 3.8% in the phacoemulsification alone group. Within 2 years, 19.2% of eyes receiving phacoemulsification alone eventually received trabeculectomy, while 25% of eyes receiving trabeculectomy required subsequent cataract surgeries or additional surgical intervention to maintain filtration. This difference was statistically insignificant.

Potential benefits of "clear lens extraction" include lower risk of damage to the corneal endothelium with a lower ultrasound energy requirement, lower risk of complications of subsequent glaucoma surgery, and no risk of cataractous progression after future glaucoma surgery. It can be considered in patients who are significantly hyperopic or presbyopic, in view of the additional refractive benefits from intraocular lens implantation. In situations where drug reduction is a high priority, trabeculectomy may be a more suitable option.

8.6 Newly Diagnosed PAC/PACG with High IOP but No Cataract

The benefit of eliminating the mechanistic role of the crystalline lens at an earlier stage has been further studied in a multicenter randomized controlled trial—the EAGLE study, in which 155 subjects with PAC and 263 patients with PACG at age 50 or above were randomized to receive either traditional laser peripheral iridotomy or clear lens extraction as the initial therapy upon diagnosis [9]. In the clear lens extraction group, 9% received concomitant viscosynechialysis, while in the laser iridotomy group, 5% received concomitant argon laser iridoplasty. Results have shown that clear lens extraction has a greater efficacy and cost-effectiveness than did laser iridotomy as the initial treatment. The group receiving clear lens extraction had a lower mean IOP (1.18 mm Hg lower), lower percentage of subjects requiring topical glaucoma medications (21% versus 61%), a lower percentage of subjects requiring glaucoma surgery (1 versus 24 operations), and a better quality of life score assessed with European Quality of Life-5

Dimensions questionnaire. Although lens extraction may be associated with potential severe intraoperative and postoperative complications, irreversible visual loss occurred in one participant in the clear lens extraction group as compared with three participants in the laser iridotomy group.

Above all, since "clear lens extraction" is not an established conventional treatment and there is no consensus yet on its use, informed consent and excellent rapport between physician and patient are of paramount importance before proceeding. Besides, patients have to be aware that cataract extraction in PACG eyes may be associated with higher surgical risk than with routine cataract surgery. Upon discussing the optimal surgical procedure for each individual patient, risks should be personalized and potential risks such as transient IOP spike or steroid-induced ocular hypertension after lens extraction have to be thoroughly explained. It is also important to understand that there is a possibility of preexisting trabecular meshwork damage in PACG eyes, which may limit the efficacy of IOP reduction by lens extraction alone in these eyes.

8.7 Lens Extraction in Acute Primary Angle Closure (APAC)

Argon laser peripheral iridoplasty (ALPI) or medical treatment, depending on facilities and expertise, remains the first-line intervention for patients suffering from acute primary angle closure (APAC). The role of early lens extraction as an alternative to laser peripheral iridotomy (LPI) has been studied in two randomized controlled trials [9–11]. In both of the trials, subjects were randomized to receive either early phacoemulsification or LPI after medically aborted APAC. Lam et al. found that treatment with LPI was associated with a significantly increased risk of subsequent IOP rise, while early phacoemulsification was associated with consistently lower IOP at all time points and required fewer medications [10]. Husain et al. showed a higher 2-year cumulative survival for the phacoemulsification group in terms of IOP control. Compared with laser iridotomy, the better IOP control after phacoemulsification in post-APAC eyes was secondary to a greater degree of opening of drainage angle and possibly flushing of the trabecular meshwork.

Despite the clear benefit of early lens extraction after APAC, the optimal timing of lens extraction after medically aborted APAC remained uncertain. Some surgeons suggest earlier lens extraction (within days) to prevent peripheral anterior synechiae (PAS) formation, but most surgeons advocate operating weeks after the resolution of the attack upon reduction of ocular inflammation and improvement of corneal clarity. To balance between PAS formation and increased operative risk, the best time window for performing lens extraction after APAC attack may be as soon as the inflammation associated with the attack has largely resolved. During the interim period, an interim LPI may be considered, especially when earlier surgery would not be possible because of logistical constraints. Although a previous trial demonstrated that the endothelial cell count did not differ significantly between LPI and phacoemulsification in this subgroup, one must consider the combined effect of the two sequential procedures if this happens.

8.8 Other IOP Lowering Procedures to be Combined with Lens Extraction in PACG

Lens extraction also provides a good opportunity where additional glaucoma procedures can be performed with the corneal wound created during lens extraction. Examples of such include combining cataract extraction with goniosynechialysis (GSL) and endocyclophotocoagulation (ECP). Combining GSL with phacoemulsification has certain advantages, including better visualization and access to the drainage angle intraoperatively, better IOP/drug reduction, a lower possibility of recurrent angle closure and PAS formation, as well as the elimination of the risk of lens damage or cataract formation after the surgery (Fig. 8.2). Combining

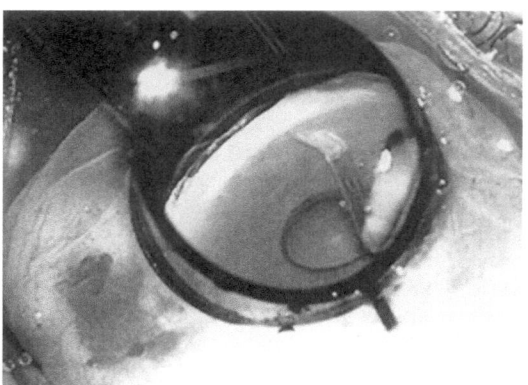

Fig. 8.2 Legend Text: During goniosynechiolysis, the angle can be visualized using a Swan Jacob direct gonio lens. Visible PAS can be broken down by pushing the peripheral iris down gently with a flat spatula inserted via a paracentesis wound. Caution is taken not to damage the iris or induce iridodialysis

ECP with lens extraction allows safe and easy access to the ciliary process with no requirement for additional incisional wound. Apart from reducing aqueous production, ECP has also been postulated to impose additional IOP lowering effect by widening anterior chamber angles, particularly in PACG eyes, by shrinking ciliary processes. A case series of five patients using intraoperative anterior segment OCT has shown a significant widening of the anterior chamber angle in eyes with plateau iris syndrome after combined phacoemulsification and ECP as compared to phacoemulsification alone [12].

8.9 Tackling Specific Operative Risks and Complications During Lens Extraction

8.9.1 Preoperative

High IOP should be adequately controlled before any surgical intervention. In selected cases, systemic acetazolamide or mannitol may be required. Corneal endothelial status should be evaluated using specular microscopy upon clinical examination and particularly in cases after acute primary angle closure or previous difficult or multiple laser procedures. Preoperative miotics should be terminated with IOP monitoring a week before surgery.

8.9.2 Intraoperative

Main surgical wound using three-step incisions and tight-angled side port paracentesis will help prevent iris prolapse. Small pupil can be tackled using various techniques, including Kuglen iris hooks, iris retractors, or Malyugin ring (Fig. 8.3). Specialized, heavy-weighted viscoelastics (such as Healon GV/5) can be used to maintain the anterior chamber during capsulorhexis, as it helps to tamponade the anterior bulging curvature of the lens, as well as prevent iris movement. High lens vault may increase the risk of runaway capsulorhexis; therefore, surgeons should take caution in maintaining a centripetal force and may require a second instrument to depress the lens. Excessive hydrodissection should be avoided as it might induce iris prolapse and, in extreme cases, inadvertent posterior capsule blowout with drop nucleus. Adequate hydrodelineation is very

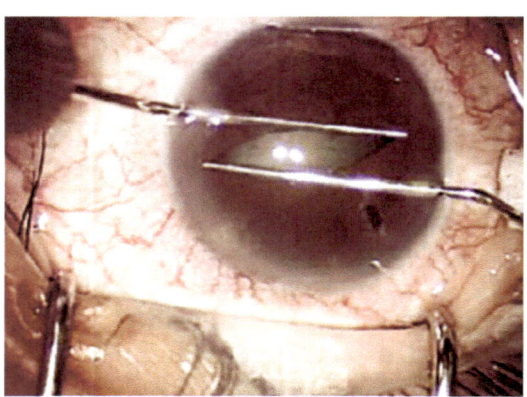

Fig. 8.3 Legend Text: Small pupil is not uncommonly encountered in patient with PACG. Kuglen hooks can be used to enlarge the pupil intraoperatively. Alternatively, iris retractors or Malyugin ring can be employed

helpful in cases with small pupil and large lens. During phacoemulsification, extra anterior chamber pressurization may be necessary to maintain the anterior chamber and to prevent endothelial damage. After implanting the intraocular lens, viscoelastics should be removed thoroughly to prevent a postoperative IOP spike. Intracameral miotics can be instilled to reverse pupil dilatation and prevent immediate peripheral anterior synechiae formation.

8.9.3 Postoperative

Additional intraoperative iris maneuvers require additional topical steroid therapy to control ocular inflammation and prevent the development of cystoid macular edema. For patients with advanced glaucomatous damage, oral acetazolamide is a good option to prevent overnight IOP spike and wipeout. Upon follow-up, surgeons should be aware of possible malignant glaucoma in this subset of patients which may require immediate YAG hyaloidotomy or vitrectomy combined with iridectomy, hyaloidectomy, and zonulectomy [13].

8.10 Conclusion

Lens extraction has a specific role in treating angle closure glaucoma. It should be considered as one of the treatment options in PACG eyes with cataracts, medically uncontrolled PACG eyes, as well as in APAC eyes after abortion of the acute episode. Concomitant filtration surgery may be considered if drug reduction is a top priority, but surgical complications should be thoroughly discussed with patients. Other adjunctive IOP-lowering procedures such as GSL or ECP can also be combined with lens extraction in suitable candidates to achieve maximal IOP lowering.

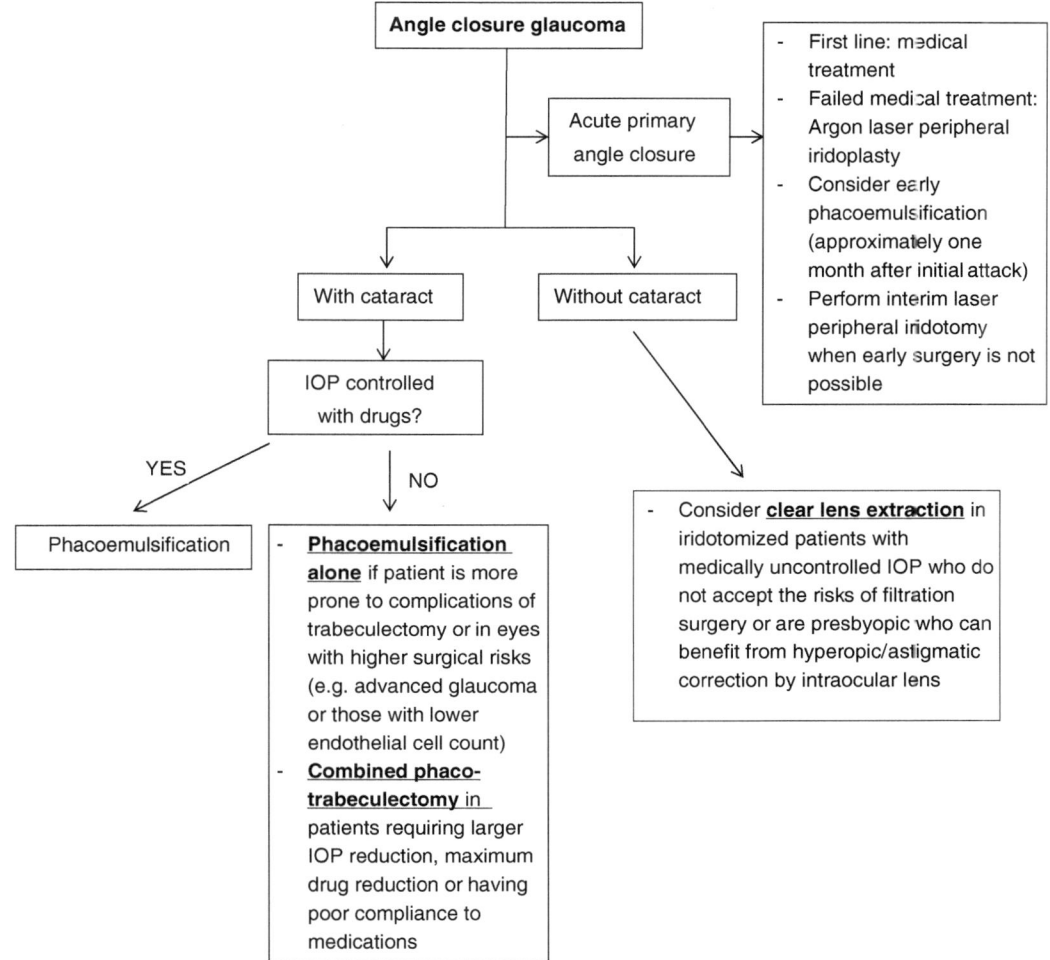

Algorithm 8.1 Cataract/Clear lens extraction as treatment strategy for angle closure and angle closure glaucoma (Abbreviations: *AC* angle closure, *ACG* angle closure glaucoma, *IOP* intraocular pressure)

An algorithm for considering cataract or clear lens extraction as a treatment strategy in angle closure diseases is provided (Algorithm 8.1).

References

1. Deng BL, Jiang C, Ma B, et al. Surgical treatment for primary angle-closure glaucoma: a meta-analysis. Int Ophthalmol. 2011;4(3):223–7.

2. Tham CC, Kwong YY, Leung DY, et al. Phacoemulsification versus combined phacotrabeculectomy in medically uncontrolled chronic angle closure glaucoma with cataracts. Ophthalmology. 2009;116(4):725–31.

3. Hansapinyo L, Choy BNK, Lai JSM, et al. Phacoemulsification versus phacotrabeculectomy in primary angle-closure glaucoma with cataract: long term clinical outcomes. J Glaucoma 2019 Nov 6; 29:15. https://doi.org/10.1097/IJG.0000000000001397. Epub ahead of print.

4. Lai JS, Tham CC, Chan JC. The clinical outcomes of cataract extraction by phacoemulsification in eyes with primary angle-closure glaucoma (PACG) and coexisting cataract: a prospective case series. J Glaucoma. 2006;15(1):47–52.

5. Tham CC, Leung DY, Kwong YY, Li FC, Lam DS. Effects of phacoemulsification versus combined phaco-trabeculectomy on drainage angle status in primary angle closure glaucoma (PACG). Glaucoma. 2010;19(2):119–23.

6. Tham CCY, Kwong YYY, Leung DYL, Lam SW, Li FCH, Chiu TYH, Chan JCH, Lam DSC, Lai JSM. Phacoemulsification vs phacotrabeculectomy in chronic angle-closure glaucoma with cataract complications. Arch Ophthalmol. 2010;128(3):303–11.

7. Man X, Chan NC, Baig N, et al. Anatomical effects of clear lens extraction by phacoemulsification versus trabeculectomy on anterior chamber drainage angle in primary angle-closure glaucoma (PACG) patients. Graefes Arch Clin Exp Ophthalmol. 2015;253: 773–8.

8. Tham CC, Kwong YY, Baig N, Leung DY, Li FC, Lam DS. Phacoemulsification versus trabeculectomy in medically uncontrolled chronic angle-closure glaucoma without cataract. Ophthalmology. 2013;120(1):62–7.

9. Azuara-Blanco A, Burr J, Ramsay C, et al., EAGLE Study Group. Effectiveness of early lens extraction for the treatment of primary angle-closure glaucoma (EAGLE): a randomised controlled trial. Lancet 2016;388:1389–1397.

10. Lam DS, Leung DY, Tham CC, et al. Randomized trial of early phacoemulsification versus peripheral iridotomy to prevent intraocular pressure rise after acute primary angle closure. Ophthalmology. 2008;115(7):1134–40.

11. Husain R, Gazzard G, Aung T, et al. Initial management of acute primary angle closure: a randomized trial comparing phacoemulsification with laser peripheral iridotomy. Ophthalmology. 2012;119:2274–81.

12. Pathak Ray V, Puri V, Peguda HK. Intra-operative ASOCT determined changes in angle recess in plateau iris syndrome post phaco alone and post phaco-endocycloplasty. Graefes Arch Clin Exp Ophthalmol. 2019 Mar;257(3):663–4.

13. Ruben S, Tsai J, Hitchings RA. Malignant glaucoma and its management. Br J Ophthalmol. 1997;81(2):163–7.

Sieh Yean Kiew, Rahat Husain, and Tin Aung

Abstract

One of the barriers to maintaining optimal intraocular pressure (IOP) control in angle closure disease is the formation of peripheral anterior synechiae (PAS). Conceptually, surgical removal of synechiae should reopen the angle and restore trabecular outflow, thus improving IOP control. In this chapter, we review the rationale, history of, and evidence for and against goniosynechialysis as a procedure in the management of synechial angle closure.

Keywords

Peripheral anterior synechiae ·
Goniosynechialysis · Primary angle closure
Primary angle closure glaucoma

S. Y. Kiew · R. Husain
Singapore National Eye Centre and Singapore Eye
Research Institute, Singapore, Singapore

Ophthalmology and Visual Sciences Academic
Clinical Program, Duke-NUS Medical School,
Singapore, Singapore

T. Aung (✉)
Singapore National Eye Centre and Singapore Eye
Research Institute, Singapore, Singapore

Ophthalmology and Visual Sciences Academic
Clinical Program, Duke-NUS Medical School,
Singapore, Singapore

Yong Loo Lin School of Medicine, National
University of Singapore, Singapore, Singapore

9.1   Background

Primary angle closure glaucoma (PACG) accounts for 25% of glaucoma worldwide, but is responsible for 50% of glaucoma-related blindness around the world [1]. The spectrum of primary angle closure disease ranges from primary angle closure suspect (PACS, ≥180 degrees of appositional iridotrabecular contact, in the absence of synechiae and with normal intraocular pressure (IOP)), primary angle closure (PAC, ≥180 degrees of iridotrabecular contact with peripheral anterior synechiae and/or raised IOP), of which acute primary angle closure is a subset, to primary angle closure glaucoma (glaucomatous optic neuropathy in the presence of ≥180 degrees of angle closure).

A variety of underlying mechanisms may play a role in PACG (Table 9.1 summarizes the mechanisms of angle closure as described by Ritch and Lowe in 1996 [2]).

Chronic appositional closure may lead to the formation of peripheral anterior synechiae (PAS)—permanent adhesions between the iris and trabecular meshwork. Conceptually, surgical removal of PAS at the time of cataract surgery should reopen the angle. Although the use of ophthalmic viscosurgical devices (OVD) during cataract surgery may break some iridotrabecular adhesions, cataract surgery alone does not fully eliminate PAS. Studies have shown that up to 32% of patients undergoing phacoemulsification

Table 9.1 Mechanisms of angle closure [2]

I	Relative pupillary block
II	Plateau iris
III	Lens-induced angle closure
IV	Forces posterior to the lens (e.g. aqueous misdirection syndrome, choroidal effusion)

surgery alone still have PAS with or without raised IOP post-operatively [3].

9.2 Goniosynechialysis: Technique and Rationale

Campbell and Vela in 1984 [4] first described goniosynechialysis as a treatment for synechial angle closure, using an irrigating cyclodialysis spatula to maintain the anterior chamber and to perform the lysis under direct visualization. In a case series, they described an 80% success rate (resolution of PAS) in cases where synechiae had been present for 1 year or less [4]. Since then, goniosynechialysis has been investigated extensively in the literature. Initial studies were promising, showing a significant reduction in IOP post-operatively, with some early reports suggesting that this procedure may be an alternative to trabeculectomy in patients with PACG [5–7].

Modern goniosynechialysis is performed either alone, or more commonly in combination with phacoemulsification surgery (phacoemulsification with goniosynechialysis, or phaco-GSL). After deepening the anterior chamber either by the use of cohesive OVD or by means of an anterior chamber maintainer, a blunt instrument such as a cyclodialysis spatula, iris repositor, or intraocular forceps such as the Ahmed micrograsper is used to gently press down on the peripheral iris, manually breaking the PAS (Fig. 9.1). Postoperatively, pilocarpine drops or argon laser iridoplasty are sometimes used to reduce the risk of reformation of PAS [8].

Goniosynechialysis is attractive for a variety of reasons. Firstly, anterior segment imaging studies have shown restoration of an anatomically open angle, with widening of all angle

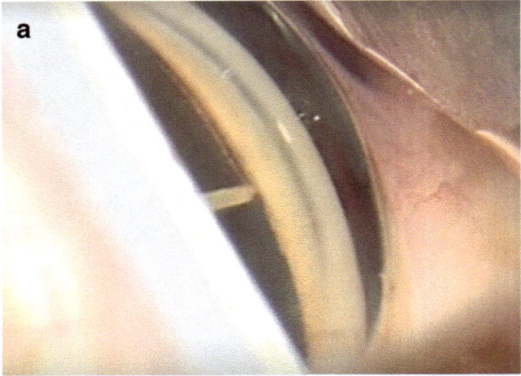

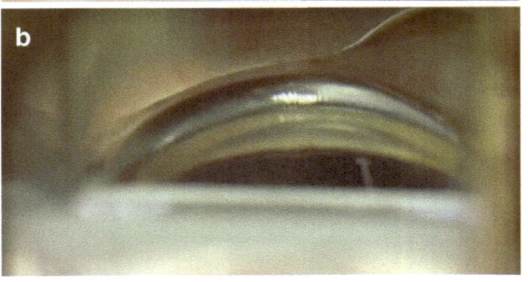

Fig. 9.1 Goniosynechialysis performed using (**a**) a cyclodialysis spatula, visualized using a Mori lens; (**b**) a goniosynechialysis spatula with a T-shaped head, visualized using a Mori lens. Pictures courtesy of Dr. Shamira Perera and Dr. Rahat Husain from Singapore National Eye Centre, reproduced with permission

parameters following phaco-GSL, compared to phacoemulsification surgery alone [9]. Beyond anatomical improvement, tonographic outflow facility studies have demonstrated improvement in aqueous outflow following phaco-GSL, significantly more than in eyes undergoing phacoemulsification alone [10]. Goniosynechialysis is minimally invasive and conjunctival-sparing, without compromising the chances of a future filtering procedure. When compared to traditional filtering procedures such as a trabeculectomy, goniosynechialysis has a significantly more favourable safety profile, with fewer potentially sight-threatening complications [6] (Table 9.2).

Furthermore, it is relatively simple and quick to perform, without requiring specialized instruments and can easily be combined with other procedures such as phacoemulsification surgery.

Table 9.2 Safety profile and complications of goniosynechialysis as compared to trabeculectomy

Potential complications	Trabeculectomy	Goniosynechialysis
Suprachoroidal/expulsive haemorrhage	Can occur	Unlikely
Late blebitis/endophthalmitis	Can occur	Unlikely
Hypotony	Can occur	Unlikely
Wound leak	Can occur	Unlikely
Aqueous misdirection	Can occur	Unlikely
IOP spike	Less likely	Can occur
Hyphaema	Can occur	Can occur
Inflammation	Can occur	Can occur

9.3   Goniosynechialysis: The Evidence

Since its first description by Campbell and Vela in 1984, there have been a number of studies investigating the results of goniosynechialysis as an IOP-lowering procedure. Early reports from the 1990s reported a drastic reduction in IOP following goniosynechialysis, with up to 26 mm Hg mean IOP reduction in patients with synechial closure of less than 6 months duration [5, 6, 11]. Kameda and colleagues in 2013 reported an 85–100% success rate at maintaining 'optimal' IOP control [7] following goniosynechialysis without the need for further surgical procedures. Zhang et al. in 2016 compared patients undergoing combined phacoemulsification and goniosynechialysis to those undergoing trabeculectomy and found comparable results at 12 months [12].

Many of these studies reported the effects of combined phaco-GSL; however, we know from existing literature that phacoemulsification (or lens removal surgery) alone has a significant IOP-lowering effect in angle closure disease [13–15]. A number of randomized controlled trials (RCTs) have been carried out comparing combined phaco-GSL to phacoemulsification alone in order to determine how much of the IOP-lowering effect seen in these procedures can be directly attributed to the goniosynechialysis procedure; the results of these are summarized in Table 9.3. While earlier RCTs [9, 10] favoured phaco-GSL over phacoemulsification alone, a meta-analysis performed by Wang et al. in 2019 [19] pooling data from seven published RCTs showed no significant difference in IOP-lowering effect or number of medications required between phacoemulsification alone and combined phaco-GSL (although Wang et al. also included in their analysis three RCTs where synechiae were broken using injection of OVD alone, or viscogonioplasty, instead of manual lysis of synechiae). Recently, two larger RCTs comparing phacoemulsification alone to phaco-GSL have been published: Husain et al. [17] studied patients with PAC or PACG and at least 90 degrees of synechial angle closure, 35 of whom were randomized to phacoemulsification alone and 33 to phaco-GSL. They found no significant differences between the groups in IOP reduction, number of IOP-lowering medications, IOP control or degree of residual PAS at 12 months postoperatively. Angmo et al. [18] examined a cohort of patients with mild-moderate PACG with at least 180 degrees of PAS and suboptimal IOP control despite maximally tolerated medical therapy. Of these, 30 were randomized to phacoemulsification alone, and 34 to phaco-GSL. They reported a significant reduction in IOP in both groups and widening of angle parameters on ASOCT at 6 months, with no statistically significant differences between groups; in fact contrary to previous reports, in this study more IOP-lowering medications were required in the phaco-GSL group than in the phacoemulsification group to maintain optimal IOP. The results from these two recent RCTs confirm the findings of Wang et al., that there may not be an advantage of phaco-GSL over phacoemulsification alone.

The major criticism of goniosynechialysis is that mechanical relief of PAS alone with restoration of a grossly open angle does not guarantee restoration of trabecular outflow. While PAS initially form on the inner surface of the trabecular

Table 9.3 Comparison of outcomes following phacoemulsification and combined phaco-GSL surgery from reported studies in the literature

Author, date	Number of patients	Follow-up duration (months)	Reduction in IOP (mmHg)		PAS reduction (degrees)		Notes
			Phaco	Phaco-GSL	Phaco	Phaco-GSL	
Lee et al. [16]	30 (15 randomized to phaco alone, 15 to phaco-GSL)	6	2.33	4.54	119	114	Both groups had a significant reduction in IOP and number of medications, no difference between phaco versus phaco-GSL groups in amount of residual PAS, post-operative IOP or number of IOP-lowering medications used
Shao et al. [9]	43 (20 randomized to phaco alone, 23 to phaco-GSL)	6	7.05	8.47	NR	NR	Better IOP control on fewer IOP-lowering medications in phaco-GSL group
Rodrigues et al. [10]	23 (10 randomized to phaco alone, 13 to phaco-GSL)	6	5.4	12.6	22.5	138.5	More significant reduction in IOP in phaco-GSL group than phaco alone, with fewer IOP-lowering medications required in phaco-GSL group.
Husain et al. [17]	68 (35 from phaco group, 33 phaco-GSL)	12	7.9	7.1	91	136	No significant difference between groups in IOP, number of medications or control at 12 months
Angmo et al. [18]	64 (30 randomized to phaco alone, 34 to phaco-GSL)	6	16.31	17.51	NR	NR	More IOP-lowering medications required in phaco-GSL group compared to phaco group to maintain optimal IOP at 6 months

Abbreviations: *phaco* phacoemulsification surgery, *phaco-GSL* combined phacoemulsification surgery with goniosynechialysis, *IOP* intraocular pressure, *mmHg* millimetres of mercury, *PAS* peripheral anterior synechiae, *NR* not reported

meshwork, scanning electron microscopy studies have shown that chronic PACG leads to irreversible changes within the meshwork ultrastructure with fewer trabecular spaces and fused trabecular beams, even in areas without PAS [20]. Histological studies have demonstrated occlusion of Schlemm's canal in PACG eyes [21], thus simply opening the angle alone may not necessarily restore flow due to chronic microscopic damage to the trabecular meshwork and Schlemm's canal. Furthermore, PAS may reform following goniosynechialysis—not only in patients with residual angle crowding but even in patients who have had goniosynechialysis combined with cataract surgery [17].

There is some evidence that goniosynechialysis may be more effective in patients with recent-onset PAS [22]; this suggests that there may possibly be a small subset of patients with recent onset of synechial closure in whom this procedure may still be beneficial, for example in those with a recent acute attack of angle closure, or with documented recent progression of synechial closure with raised IOP, and mild to moderate glaucoma. However, duration of PAS is notoriously difficult to ascertain with any accuracy; even in cases of acute primary angle closure there is no surety that the PAS formed at that time point because of the phenomenon of 'acute on chronic' disease.

One study has shown that laser iridoplasty reduces reformation of PAS post-goniosynechialysis [8]; whether this confers any additional clinical benefit following phaco-GSL in terms of sustained or larger IOP reduction however has yet to be proven. Where PAS is chronic or long-standing, in theory, a goniotomy procedure in combination with phaco-GSL might improve outcomes by allowing aqueous access to the outer trabecular meshwork or Schlemm's canal, bypassing the damaged inner trabecular meshwork, but there is no good evidence at the moment to recommend this approach.

9.4 Conclusions

There is now robust evidence that goniosynechialysis does not confer any additional benefit over phacoemulsification surgery alone in terms of IOP reduction, control and medication requirements in patients with synechial PACG. However, in selected cases of recent onset of PAS, goniosynechialysis may still be useful in opening the angle and reducing IOP. This finding, namely that phaco-GSL works very well for some patients and not for others may simply be reflective of the functionality of the trabecular meshwork. If functionality could somehow be determined pre-operatively, then manual removal of the physical obstruction of the trabecular meshwork (i.e. removal of PAS via GSL) would most likely result in good IOP lowering. Determining trabecular meshwork functionality before surgery is embarked would be very useful and is where future research in this area should be directed.

References

1. Foster PJ. The epidemiology of primary angle closure and associated glaucomatous optic neuropathy. Semin Ophthalmol. 2002;17(2):50–8.
2. Ritch R, Lowe R. Angle closure glaucoma: mechanisms and epidemiology. In: Ritch R, Shields M, Krupin T, editors. The Glaucomas. 2nd ed. St Louis: Mosby; 1996. p. 801–19.
3. Aung T, Tow SL, Yap EY, Chan SP, Seah SK. Trabeculectomy for acute primary angle closure. Ophthalmology. 2000;107(7):1298–302.
4. Campbell DG, Vela A. Modern goniosynechialysis for the treatment of synechial angle-closure glaucoma. Ophthalmology. 1984;91(9):1052–60.
5. Shingleton BJ, Chang MA, Bellows AR, Thomas JV. Surgical goniosynechialysis for angle-closure glaucoma. Ophthalmology. 1990;97(5):551–6.
6. Tanihara H, Nishiwaki K, Nagata M. Surgical results and complications of goniosynechialysis. Graefes Arch Clin Exp Ophthalmol. 1992;230(4):309–13.
7. Kameda T, Inoue T, Inatani M, Tanihara H. Long-term efficacy of goniosynechialysis combined with phaco-emulsification for primary angle closure. Graefes Arch Clin Exp Ophthalmol. 2013;251(3):825–30.
8. Tanihara H, Nagata M. Argon-laser gonioplasty following goniosynechialysis. Graefes Arch Clin Exp Ophthalmol. 1991;229(6):505–7.
9. Shao T, Hong J, Xu J, Le Q, Wang J Qian S. Anterior chamber angle assessment by anterior-segment optical coherence tomography after phacoemulsification with or without Goniosynechialysis in patients with primary angle closure Glaucoma. J Glaucoma. 2015;24(9):647–55.
10. Rodrigues IA, Alaghband P, Beltran Agullo L, et al. Aqueous outflow facility after phacoemulsification with or without goniosynechialysis in primary angle closure: a randomised controlled study. Br J Ophthalmol. 2017;101(7):879–85.
11. Teekhasaenee C, Ritch R. Combined phacoemulsification and goniosynechialysis for uncontrolled chronic angle-closure glaucoma after acute angle-closure glaucoma. Ophthalmology 1999;106(4):669–674; discussion 674–665.
12. Zhang H, Tang G, Liu J. Effects of phacoemulsification combined with Goniosynechialysis on primary angle-closure Glaucoma. J Glaucoma. 2016;25(5):e499–503.
13. Thomas R, Walland M, Thomas A, Mengersen K. Lowering of intraocular pressure after phacoemulsification in primary open-angle and angle-closure Glaucoma: a Bayesian analysis. Asia Pac J Ophthalmol (Phila). 2016;5(1):79–84.
14. Moghimi S, Lin S. Role of phacoemulsification in angle closure glaucoma. Eye Sci. 2011;26(3):121–31.
15. Tham CC, Kwong YY, Leung DY, et al. Phacoemulsification versus combined phacotrabeculectomy in medically uncontrolled chronic angle closure glaucoma with cataracts. Ophthalmology. 2009;116(4):725–731, 731.e721–723.
16. Lee CK, Rho SS, Sung GJ, et al. Effect of Goniosynechialysis during phacoemulsification on IOP in patients with medically well-controlled chronic angle-closure Glaucoma. J Glaucoma. 2015;24(6):405–9.
17. Husain R, Do T, Lai J, et al. Efficacy of phacoemulsification alone vs phacoemulsification with Goniosynechialysis in patients with primary angle-closure disease: a randomized clinical trial. JAMA Ophthalmol. 2019;137:1107.
18. Angmo D, Shakrawal J, Gupta B, Yadav S, Pandey R, Dada T. Comparative evaluation of phacoemulsification alone versus phacoemulsification with Goniosynechialysis in primary angle-closure

Glaucoma: a randomized controlled trial. Ophthalmol Glaucoma. 2019;2:346.

19. Wang N, Jia SB. Phacoemulsification with or without goniosynechialysis for angle-closure glaucoma: a global meta-analysis based on randomized controlled trials. Int J Ophthalmol. 2019;12(5): 826–33.

20. Sihota R, Goyal A, Kaur J, Gupta V, Nag TC. Scanning electron microscopy of the trabecular meshwork: understanding the pathogenesis of pri-

mary angle closure glaucoma. Indian J Ophthalmol. 2012;60(3):183–8.

21. Hamanaka T, Kasahara K, Takemura T. Histopathology of the trabecular meshwork and Schlemm's canal in primary angle-closure glaucoma. Invest Ophthalmol Vis Sci. 2011;52(12):8849–61.

22. Tian T, Li M, Pan Y, Cai Y, Fang Y. The effect of phacoemulsification plus goniosynechialysis in acute and chronic angle closure patients with extensive goniosynechiae. BMC Ophthalmol. 2019;19(1):65.

Filtration Surgery and Glaucoma Drainage Devices in PACG

10

M. Nazrul Islam

Abstract

Surgical treatment of Angle Closure Glaucoma (ACG) is an essential part of the glaucoma patient care. The effectiveness of the different surgical treatment options depends on the anatomy of angle closure eyes. Filtration surgery (Trabeculectomy) with few modifications is commonly being done for ACG. This surgery is different in some steps than those for open angle glaucoma. The surgery also depends upon some key factors such as the level of intraocular pressure (IOP) control with medical treatment and the presence of cataract. The outcome of filtration surgery for angle closure glaucoma usually less favourable in comparison to open angle glaucoma. Surgical treatment of ACG has a higher risk of filtration failure. The filtration surgery or Trabeculectomy increases the chance of shallowing of the anterior chamber. This type of surgery usually increases the risk of malignant glaucoma and the formation of cataract. On the other hand, Glaucoma Drainage Devices (GDD) are useful in some refractory ACG and in the failed filtration surgery cases.

Keywords

Angle closure glaucoma · Filtration surgery Trabeculectomy · Shallow anterior chamber Glaucoma drainage devices

10.1 Introduction

It has been estimated by HA Quigley and AT Broman that there were 60.5 million people with Open Angle Glaucoma (OAG) and ACG in 2010, increasing to 79.6 million by 2020, and of these, 74% have OAG. Women comprise 55% of OAG, 70% of ACG. Asians represent 47% of all glaucoma and 87% of those with ACG [1].

Angle Closure is recently classified as Primary Angle Closure Suspect (PACS), Primary Angle Closure (PAC) and Primary Angle Closure Glaucoma (PACG) [2] Management of patients with angle closure disease depends on different type of clinical stage, e.g. PACS, PAC or PACG and its underlying pathophysiology. We use different treatment options for PACG which may be medical, laser or surgical, with some challenges in the treatment of PACG. Two important challenges are to prevent the angle closure and to prevent progression of the glaucomatous optic neuropathy. Number of surgical procedures with different potentialities is done for the treatment of this kind of glaucoma.

M. N. Islam (✉)
Bangladesh Eye Hospital and Institute (BEHI), Dhaka, Bangladesh

© Springer Nature Singapore Pte Ltd. 2021
C. C. Y. Tham (ed.), *Primary Angle Closure Glaucoma (PACG)*,
https://doi.org/10.1007/978-981-15-8120-5_10

10.1.1 Common Surgery in Angle Closure Glaucoma

- External procedures:
  - Filtration surgery/trabeculectomy
  - Non-penetrating surgery (NPS)
  - Viscocanalostomy
  - Glaucoma drainage devices (GDD)
  - Laser cyclophotocoagulation
- Internal procedures:
  - Goniosynechialysis
  - Viscogonioplasty
  - Goniopuncture

10.2 Filtration Surgery/ Trabeculectomy in PACG

Trabeculectomy or the partial thickness scleral flap over the fistula was first popularized by Cairns in 1968 [3]. With some modifications, this is the most common surgical procedure in the Angle Closure Glaucoma. But unlike open angle glaucoma, many times we find the difficulties in ACG such as:

(a) Anterior chamber (AC) usually very shallow.
(b) Intraoperative Floppy Iris Syndrome.
(c) Difficult to maintain AC.
(d) Peripheral anterior Synechia (PAS) is common.

Though Trabeculectomy in ACG is performed almost similarly as we do it for open angle glaucoma, but there are some variations in ACG:

(a) We must do a surgical peripheral iridectomy (PI) at the time of trabeculectomy.
(b) Adjunctive antifibrotic agents viz. antimetabolite (Mitomycin C/5 Fluorouracil) and/or anti-vascular endothelial growth factor (VEGF) is to be used with trabeculectomy to achieve a low-target IOP and decrease failure rate.
(c) In case of an acute attack of angle closure if IOP control remains suboptimal despite laser and medical treatment Trabeculectomy alone or combined with cataract, surgery can be considered.

In General Filtration Surgery in the ACG Needs

(a) Thicker superficial scleral flap, more than half thickness.
(b) Tighter closure of the scleral flap.
(c) Use of releasable tight sutures.
(d) AC should be formed by BSS or air.
(e) Surgery should be performed under surface or subconjunctival anaesthesia, so that there will be less ocular pressure.
(f) Viscogonioplasty can be helpful in cataract surgery or in combined cataract and filtration surgery [4].
(g) Non-penetrating surgery, e.g. non-penetrating deep sclerectomy (NPDS) is helpful to prevent post-operative inflammation, AC reaction and shallow anterior chamber [5].

The success rate is low in filtration surgery in the acutely inflamed eyes [6]. Some patients with nanophthalmos and very narrow angle need special attention. These very narrow hypermetropic eyes usually have short axial lengths and proportionally large lens. Surgery in these patients are prone to serious complications both during and after intraocular surgery. Common complications are per operative vitreous loss and corneal endothelial damage. Post-operative hypotony, effusions in the suprachoroidal space are common.

10.2.1 Surgical Steps

1. **Anaesthesia**

Filtration surgery is commonly done under local peribulbar anaesthesia. Usually 2% lidocaine 2 ml and 0.5% bupivacaine 2 ml is mixed and given in the floor of the orbit. In most ACG cases, my practice is sub-Tenon's anaesthesia supplemented by intracameral lidocaine if required. It does not increase the orbital pressure and there is least chance of damaging the optic nerve. Subconjunctival or sub-Tenon's anaesthesia is recommended for any type of advanced glaucoma cases.

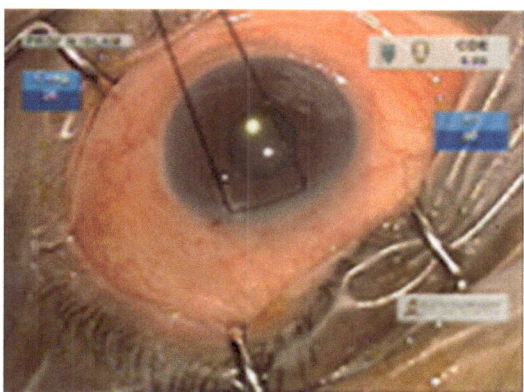

Fig. 10.1   Corneal traction suture with 6/0 silk

2. **Corneal traction suture**

Adequate surgical exposure can be obtained by a corneal traction suture. A 6/0 silk or a 6/0 vicryl traction suture is done. In the upper part of the cornea, near the superior limbus, a spatulated needle is placed through its half thickness and attached to the speculum or drape below the eye (Fig. 10.1). For the cases with subconjunctival or sub-Tenon's anaesthesia, usually the patient can cooperate to look down and the corneal traction suture is not required.

Some surgeon uses superior rectus bridle suture to expose the surgical field, but this suture may produce haemorrhage. Clotted blood may result in fibrosis in later period and failure of bleb, so it is not recommended.

3. **Antifibrotic agents**

It is used to prevent post-operative scarring or fibrosis. Per operative antifibrotic agents are used in filtration surgery including antimetabolites—MMC, 5 FU or anti-VEGF, etc.

Commonly surgeons use the microsponge soaked with 0.2–0.4 mg/cc concentration of MMC for 1–3 min. The sponge can be applied before or after making the superficial scleral flap. I use subconjunctival low-concentration MMC (0.1 cc of 0.3 mg/cc MMC diluted with 0.1 cc lidocaine) in the superior fornix and allowed to diffuse throughout by soft use of squint hook. Washing of the MMC-induced conjunctival sur-

face thoroughly by 30–50 cc BSS is done. After 5–10 min, peritomy is done either limbal based or fornix based. Multiple studies show that it does not have a significant difference in the outcome of controlling IOP [7, 8].

My preference is mostly fornix based except any scar in the limbus from previous surgery such as aphakia, pseudophakia.

4. **Cauterization**

With a bipolar wet field cautery, mild cauterization is done in the flap area.

5. **Scleral flap**

More than half-thickness lamellar scleral flap, towards the limbus, is then dissected. Scleral dissection should be not less than half thickness and forward anteriorly up to 1 mm of the peripheral cornea. This bluish-grey zone exposed is the roof of Trabecular meshwork. The scleral flap may be square, triangular or trapezoid shaped. My usual practice is making a 4 × 4 square flap (Fig. 10.3). In studies shown in regard to the long-term success rate, there is no apparent advantage of square or triangular flap [9].

In this stage, I do an oblique paracentesis by a 15-degree knife for any communication with the anterior chamber. An incision is then given at the periphery of the cornea just at the hinge of the scleral flap with the same 15-degree knife to enter the anterior chamber. The incision then widened, up to 0.5 mm of the scleral flap margins. Two radial incisions are then given posteriorly on both ends of the initial incision. The incision extends posteriorly about 1 mm, and now the flap is reflected. In case of an ideal scleral flap 2 or 3 ciliary processes are visible posteriorly.

6. **Excision of trabecular tissue**

The trabecular and peripheral corneal tissue is then excised by scissors. Now majority surgeons prefer using a Kelly Descemet's membrane scleral punch for making the fistula. My preference is to use the punch about 2/3 mm posteriorly, expecting the posterior flow [10].

7. Use of viscoelastics or air in AC

In the filtration surgery of Angle Closure Glaucoma, some surgeons use viscoelastic agents, e.g. methyl cellulose, chondroitin sulphate or sodium hyaluronate, in the anterior chamber [11]. It can reduce some complications like shallow or flat anterior chamber or hyphema in the angle closure stage of neovascular glaucoma. It reduces intraoperative hypotony. Long-time hypotony may result in suprachoroidal effusion. The complications of intracameral viscoelastics may be per operative iris prolapse and later higher post-operative IOP [11]. In this situation, I use air in the anterior chamber and after surgery; if AC is not formed then some amount of air is kept in the AC. The air is usually absorbed within 2–3 days and helps to keep the AC formed and prevents flat AC and its complications.

8. Infusion cannula

Some surgeons routinely use infusion cannula as AC maintainer. If the AC is very shallow, AC maintainer can help. It reduces the hypotony during the surgery.

9. Peripheral iridectomy (PI)

Usually, peripheral iridectomy (PI) is done in filtration surgery. Some surgeons omit this part in case of open angle glaucoma, especially with deep AC [12], but it is a must in the surgery of angle closure glaucoma. The iridectomy should be broad-based and sufficient if 2 or 3 ciliary processes are visible through PI. To avoid obstruction to the fistula made, PI should extend beyond the margins of sclerectomy.

10. Closure of scleral flap

As mentioned earlier, the scleral flap is usually half-thickness in the OAG, but in the angle closure glaucoma, the flap needs to be slightly more thicker (not more than two/third thick). Total 2–4 sutures are given in the flap and should be tighter. If required, 1 or 2 releasable sutures can be given. It helps to maintain the AC post-operatively. In the event of early post-operative higher IOP, suture can be released in the releasable suture cases after 2 weeks. Alternatively, argon/diode laser suture lysis (Fig. 10.2) can be done in the other cases between 2 and 4 weeks [13]. The primary route of external filtration is around the margins of the scleral flap. It can be examined by fluorescein angiographic studies [14].

11. Conjunctival closure

As in all types of glaucoma, watertight closure of the conjunctival flap is also required in angle closure glaucoma. Loose closure may produce wound leaking and leads to a flat AC or a flat bleb or both. This may also lead to hypotony and its complications, e.g. maculopathy, suprachoroidal effusion, etc. Many surgeons use 2–3 interrupted sutures to close the conjunctival flap, especially in the open angle glaucoma cases [14, 15]. In angle closure glaucoma, the conjunctival flap closure should be more precise, and my practice is to do horizontal running mattress suture from one end to the other [Fig. 10.3]. Absorbable suture 8/0, 9/0 or 10/0 with a fine tapered needle can be used. I use 8/0 vicryl in most of my cases.

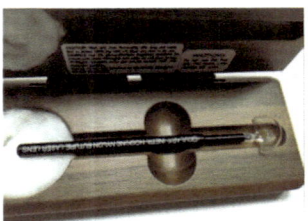 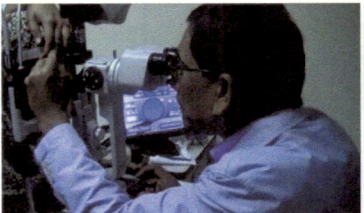 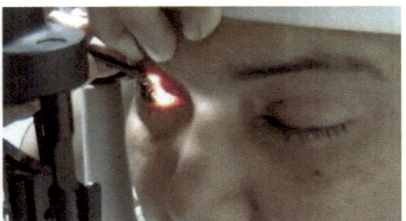

Hoskins Lens   ALSL procedure   Hoskins Lens over the suture

Fig. 10.2 Argon laser suture lysis (ALSL)

Trabeculectomy in ACG

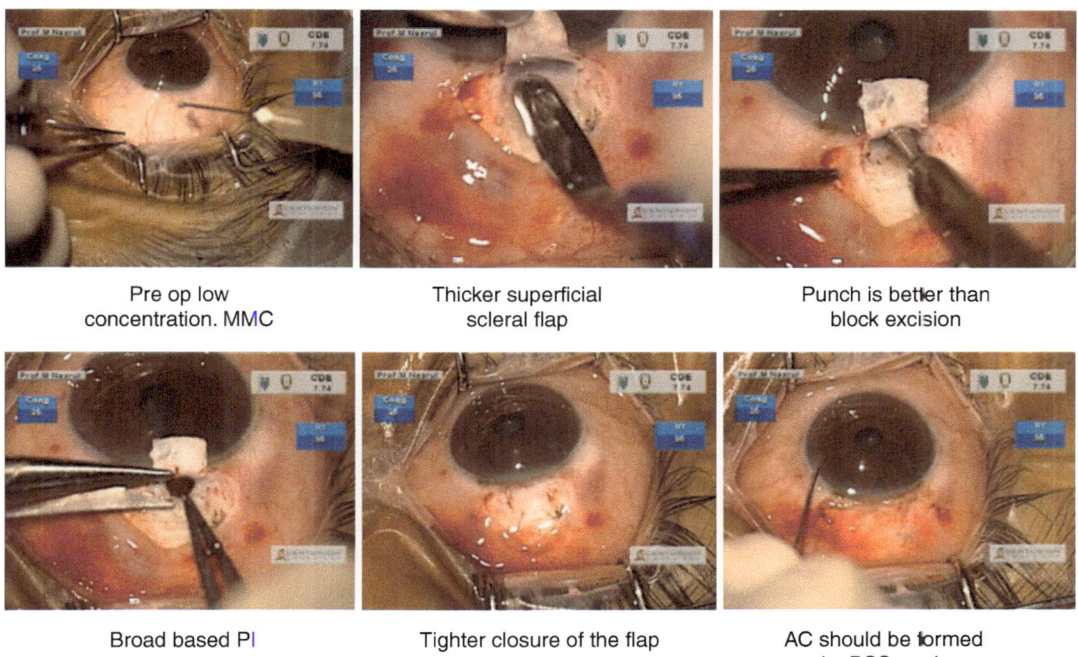

Pre op low concentration. MMC	Thicker superficial scleral flap	Punch is better than block excision
Broad based PI	Tighter closure of the flap	AC should be formed by BSS or air

Fig. 10.3 Surgical steps of trabeculectomy in ACG

After conjunctival closure, it is better to examine by fluorescein, coating the bleb surface and to see whether any bleb leak is present. If any leak is found, then further scleral flap suture or conjunctival suture or both may be needed.

10.2.2 Risk and Complications of Filtration Surgery in ACG

Filtration surgery or trabeculectomy in PACG is usually associated with a higher risk of filtration failure, hypotony, shallow anterior chamber, cataract formation, suprachoroidal haemorrhage and malignant glaucoma/aqueous misdirection [16, 17]. It is sometimes associated with the bleb leaks and blebitis. These risks are further increased by per operative use of adjunctive antimetabolite.

Cataract extraction has a deleterious effect on previous filtration surgery. It may result in a loss of the functioning filter. Tham et al. reported that 30–100% of previously functioning blebs required anti-glaucoma medications to control IOP after cataract extraction in the ACG [17].

10.2.3 Post-operative Management

Topical antibiotics should be given for 3 weeks. Usually, fourth-generation fluoroquinolone such as moxifloxacin is given 4–6 times per day for 3 weeks, and topical cycloplegic agents for 2 weeks. This drug maintains anterior chamber depth, reduces post-operative inflammation and prevents the possibility of malignant glaucoma.

Topical corticosteroids are given for a longer time up to 6–12 weeks. It reduces conjunctival scarring and have a higher success rate. Oral analgesics and sedative can be given if the patient needs. Some patients need individual post-operative care including digital bleb massage, argon laser suture lysis or bleb needling.

Nonpenetrating Procedures in ACG

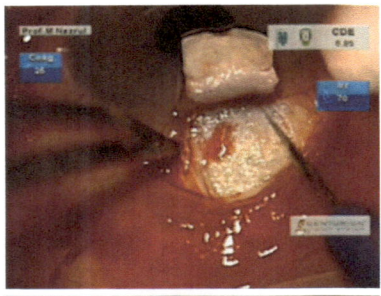 Incision for deeper scleral flap

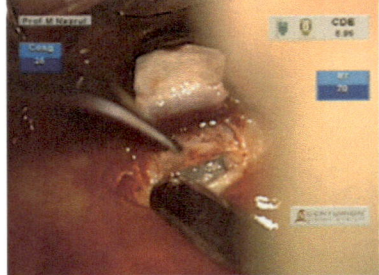 Dissecting deeper scleral flap

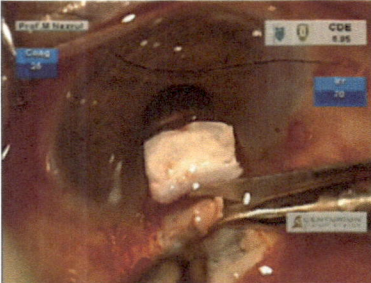 Excising deeper scleral flap

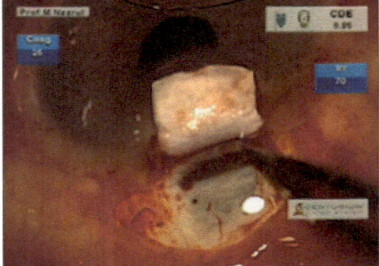 Pulling out the thin outer wall of Schelemm's canal

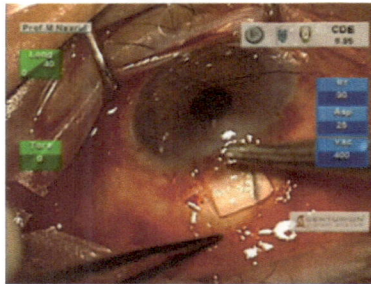 Suturing superficial scleral flap

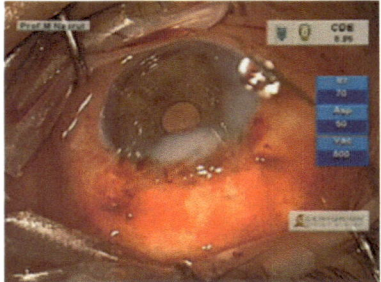 Bleb formation after the surgery

Fig. 10.4 Steps of non-penetrating deep sclerectomy (NPDS)

10.3 Trabeculectomy Versus Non-penetrating Surgeries

Non-penetrating glaucoma surgeries are also termed as non-penetrating deep sclerectomy (NPDS) or non-penetrating procedures (Fig. 10.4). The major advantage of NPDS is less complication rate. On the other hand, trabeculectomy decreases the IOP more efficiently than the non-penetrating deep sclerectomy technique in most cases [18].

NPDS may be combined with phacoemulsification in the case of ACG. It may have IOP reduction; almost similar to that can be achieved with phacoemulsification combined with filtration surgery, but with lower complication rates. Some surgeons use

CO_2 laser to do the NPDS with a higher success rate. NPDS with sclerectomy with collagen implantation has similar IOP lowering results as with trabeculectomy. In this case, post-operative complication was less. In the long term, some patients needed goniopuncture to further decrease of IOP [19, 20].

10.4 Glaucoma Drainage Devices in Angle Closure Glaucoma

Glaucoma drainage devices (GDD) or tubes are being used mostly for both open and closed angle refractory glaucoma. In some indications, e.g. neovascular angle closure glaucoma or inflammatory angle closure glaucoma, the tube may not be placed in the anterior chamber due to peripheral anterior synechia. In these situations, the tube can be placed in the posterior chamber in front of IOL if it is a case of pseudophakia. Sometimes tube is to be placed in the anterior vitreous cavity after proper vitrectomy. Currently, there is a wide variety of GDD being used. The GDD are classified as:

- **Non-valved devices:**
  - Molteno implant
  - Baerveldt
  - Aurolab aqueous drainage implant (AADI)
- **Valved devices:**
  - Ahmed glaucoma valve (AGV)

Although Ahmed clear path and Paul glaucoma implant (PGI) are two non-valved devices that have been introduced recently, still we do not have long-term results in ACG.

Glaucoma drainage device's success rate for complicated cases are from 70 to 90% to control IOP. GDD implant is also technically difficult like trabeculectomy. It may sometime produce serious complications. Glaucoma implant for ACG has been confined to those patients who had previous filtering procedures and have failed.

Some primary indications for GDD implant in the closed angle are inflammatory glaucoma, neovascular glaucoma, pseudophakic glaucoma or post-operative secondary glaucoma from retinal or corneal surgery.

In some studies, it was found that filtration surgery had poor results and was successful in only one-third of patients in the refractory glaucoma [21].

GDD used in angle closure glaucoma maybe both valved or non-valved devices. Usually, it is the surgeon's choice as to which device he or she wants to use.

10.4.1 Non-valved Open Tube Drainage Devices

1. **Molteno implant**

Molteno implant was introduced in 1969 and is the prototype drainage implant. This device has the most extensive clinical experience for a long time. Its original design was a single plate of thin acrylic with a diameter of 13 mm and a surface area of 135 mm^2. The upper surface of the plate is connected with a silicon tube. The external diameter of the tube is 0.62 mm and the internal diameter is 0.30 mm (Fig. 10.5) [22, 23].

2. **Baerveldt implant**

Baerveldt non-valved drainage implant is the most popular non-valved device. It has a large surface area of the plates with 250 mm^2 (20 mm × 13 mm) or 350 mm^2 (32 mm × 14 mm) area [24]. The implant is designed in such a way that it can be implanted through a one-quadrant conjunctival incision. A silicone tube is attached to the barium-impregnated silicone plate. The plate part of the implant is typically positioned

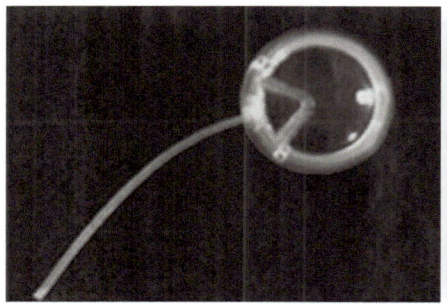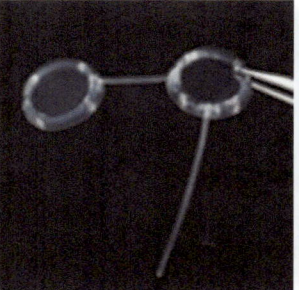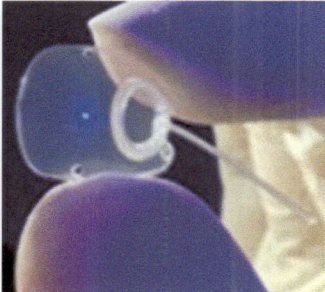

Fig. 10.5 Molteno implants Courtesy: https://www.molteno.com

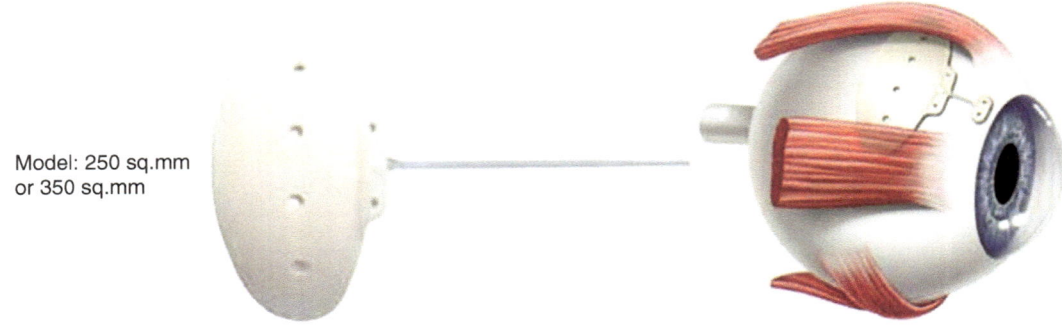

Model: 250 sq.mm
or 350 sq.mm

Fig. 10.6 Baerveldt implant

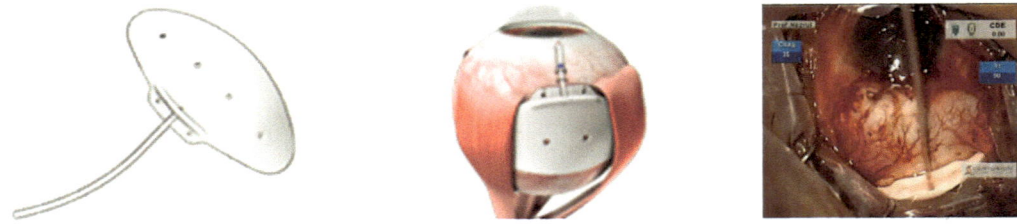

Fig. 10.7 AADI implant at superotemporal quadrant

under two rectus muscle insertions. If there is no fibrosis of the conjunctiva, the implant is usually placed in the superotemporal quadrant under the superior rectus and lateral rectus. The Baerveldt implant plate has fenestrations through which the growth of fibrous tissue occurs and helps to secure the plate (Fig. 10.6). The fibrous tissue also reduces the height of the bleb and decreases the risk for diplopia. After the first 3–6 post-operative weeks, a fibrous capsule is formed into which fluid can drain. Usually after 6 weeks, aqueous can be absorbed by the surrounding tissues, and the patient's IOP decreases.

3. **AADI—Aurolab   Aqueous   Drainage Implant**

AADI is a non-valved glaucoma drainage device. This device is designed and manufactured by Aravind Eye Care, India (Fig. 10.7). In this implant, a silicone tube is connected to a silicone plate. The surface area of the device is 350 mm^2 with a plate length of 32 mm and tube length of 35 mm [25]. Its function and surgical steps are similar to Baerveldt implant.

10.4.2 Valved or Flow Restricted Drainage Devices

Ahmad Glaucoma Valve (AGV) Implant
The Ahmed glaucoma valve implant is a popular and most commonly used valved implants in refractory glaucoma including angle closure glaucoma. Different models are in use—FP7 which has a silicone body (paediatric counterpart FP 8) and S2 which uses a propylene body (paediatric counterpart S3). For the pars plana PC7, PC8, PS2 or PS3 is used (Fig. 10.8). Aqueous outflow has less resistance through this valved device and increases resistance when the plate becomes encapsulated. The advantage of a valve mechanism in this implant is to decrease early post-operative hypotony due to resistance to the flow and to regulate the pressure within the desired range [26].

10.4.3 Surgical Techniques of GDD Implant in Angle Closure Glaucoma

Surgical techniques of GDD implant in ACG (Fig. 10.9) are similar to the technique in open

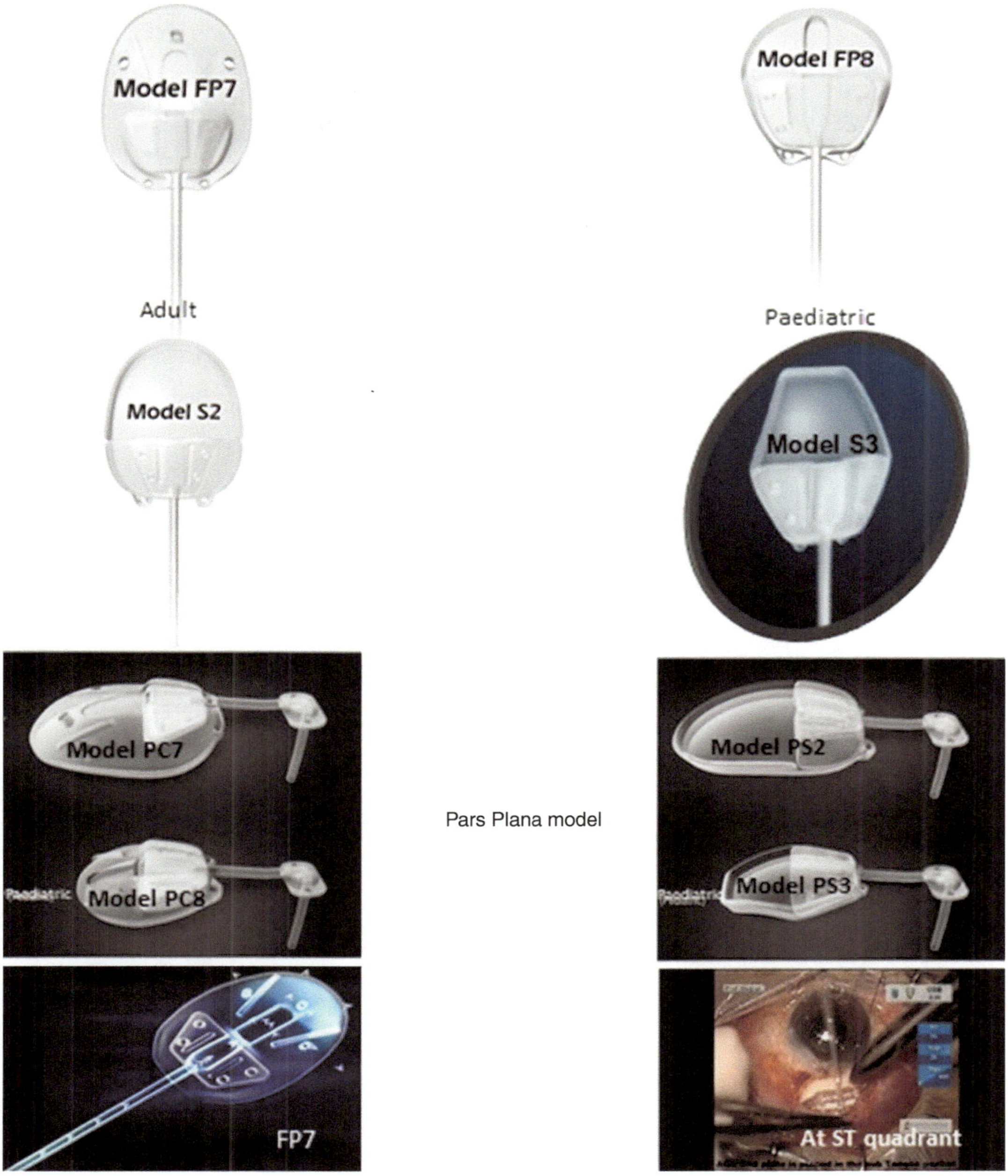

Fig. 10.8 Ahmed glaucoma valve's different common design

angle glaucoma except putting the tube in the anterior chamber. Sometimes the AC is very shallow that the tube cannot be placed in AC and then it can be placed in the sulcus in case of apseudophakic eye. In some ACG, the anterior chamber is flat, peripheral anterior synechia is

360 degree, tube can only be inserted through the pars plana to the anterior vitreous cavity after partial or complete pars plana anterior vitrectomy.

The following are the steps for the GDD implant:

GDD (AGV) – surgical steps

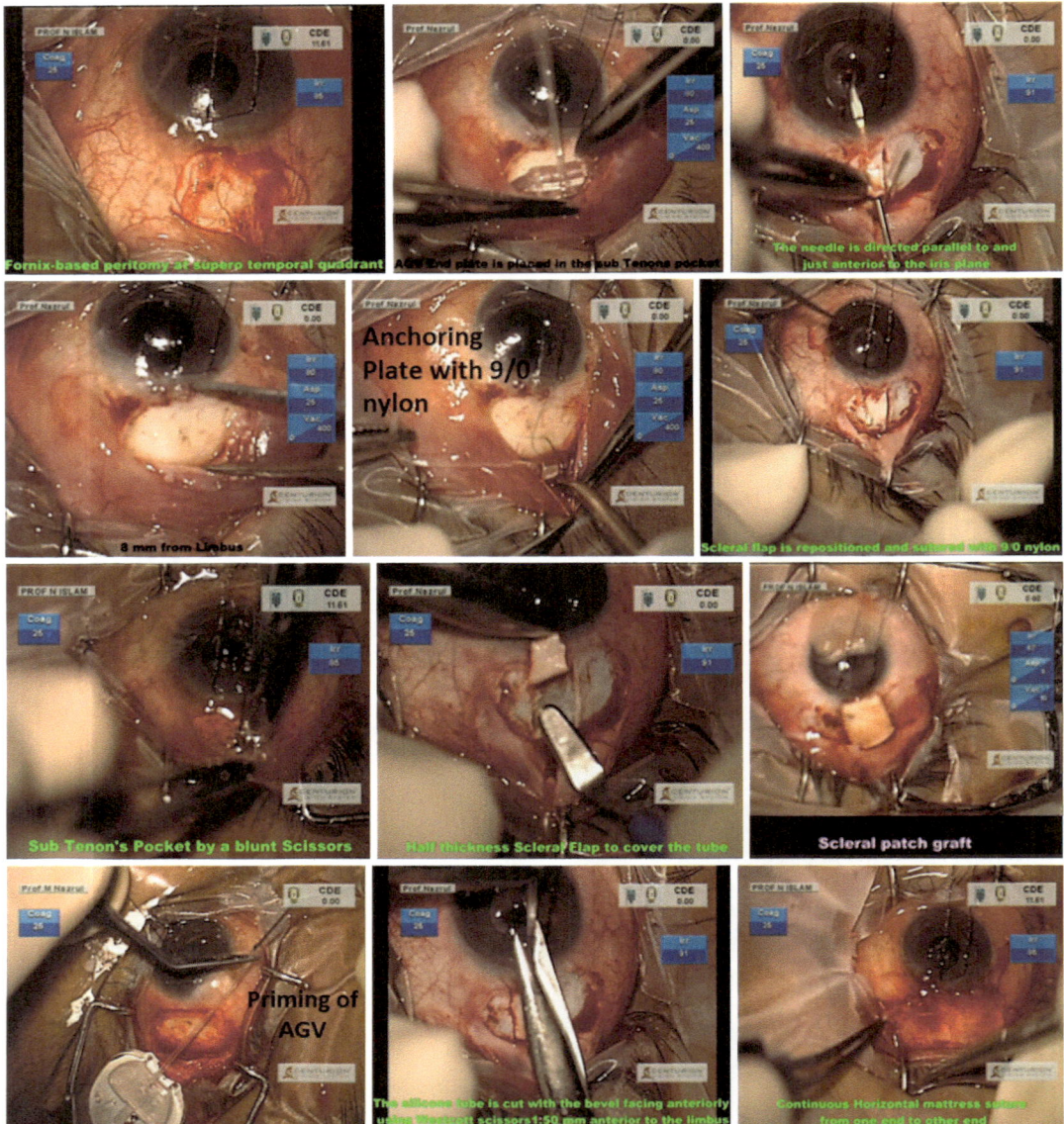

Fig. 10.9 Surgical steps of AGV implant

1. **Surgical exposure**
   - Quadrant selection: Unless fibrosis or other pathology, the AGV is usually implanted in the superotemporal quadrant. In the case of silicone oil in the anterior chamber, the inferior quadrant helps to prevent tube block by silicon oil.

   - A traction suture is needed for adequate surgical exposure. A 6-0 vicryl (polyglactin) or a 6/0 silk traction suture on a spatulated needle is commonly used. It is placed through half-thickness of the superior cornea near the limbus and attached to the eye drape or speculum beneath the eye.

- A fornix-based conjunctival incision is given. Tenons capsules can be incised separately or with conjunctiva. To improve surgical exposure, radial relaxing incisions on both sides of the conjunctival flap are given. For the non-valved open type of GDD, a squint hook is used to detect and separate the superior rectus and lateral rectus muscles on the sides of the surgical site.
2. **Valved device**
   - With Ahmed valve implant, priming should be done with a balanced salt solution (BSS) using a 27-gauge cannula. It should be ensured that the valve opens properly, and BSS passes freely. The external plate is then tucked posteriorly into the sub-Tenon space and is sutured to the sclera with non-absorbable 9/0 proline or nylon sutures through the anterior positional holes of the plate. The anterior border of the plate should be at 8–9 mm posterior to the limbus [27].
3. **Non-valve devices**
   - With non-valve devices, the tube must be occluded by 6/0 vicryl to restrict the aqueous flow. Tube occlusion should be tested by a balanced salt solution with a 30-gauge cannula.

     This tube occlusion will prevent possible early post-operative hypotony. This occlusion also prevents any drainage of aqueous for 4–6 weeks after the operation when the vicryl suture dissolves.

     The tube is then shortened with bevel up to its optimum size, and so 1.5–2 mm should remain in the anterior chamber. A paracentesis is usually required to put air, BSS or viscoelastic in the anterior chamber. Anterior chamber depth should be optimum. Excess visco will displace the iris posteriorly and may cause anatomical misplacement of tube insertion.
4. **In the anterior chamber**
   - A 23-gauge needle is used to create a needle track for the same 23-gauge AGV tube. The anterior chamber is entered by a curved needle, parallel to the iris plane. As the needle is the same size as the tube, it

creates a watertight seal. It also prevents leakage around the tube and reduces the risk of post-operative hypotony.
- To insert the tube to the anterior chamber, specially designed tube-insertion forceps can be used. I use Moorfield Forceps, which also can be used.
- The tube size in the anterior chamber should be checked. If longer than expected then resize can be done by pulling out the tube and re-inserted. The anterior chamber should be well-formed with either BSS or viscoelastic.
- The tube is then secured to the sclera by non-absorbable suture, such as 8/0, 9/0 or 10/0 nylon. I use 9/0 nylon in most of my cases.
5. **Covering of tube**
   - Covering the tube properly is an important step. Majority surgeons use preserved donor tissue over the tube. Donor sclera, processed pericardium and fascia lata are available commercially for this purpose. In most of my cases, I cover the tube under partial-thickness scleral flap. Recently I prefer short tunnel short flap (STSF) to cover the AGV tube, and then suturing the flap by 9/0 or 10/0 nylon. For non-valved tubes, I give 2–3 tube fenestrations for temporary aqueous flow before the ligatures absorb and open the tube.
   - The conjunctiva is then apposed and sutured. I do horizontal mattress suture using 8/0 vicryl sutures (Fig. 10.9).
6. **Subconjunctival medications**
   - Usually, the GDD are done under local or sub-Tenon's anaesthesia, and after completion of the surgery, subconjunctival steroids and antibiotics are injected in the opposite quadrant. Post-operative topical steroid–antibiotic and mydriatic–cycloplegic preparations are used for 4–6 weeks.

10.4.4 Complications of GDD

1. *Hypotony*: Post-operative hypotony is common in non-valved devices if the tube is not

occluded completely. For the valved device, if there is excess leaking around the tube, it may cause early post-operative hypotony. Usually, IOP increases when the fibrous capsule has developed around the external plate. Per operative high-density viscoelastics can help to prevent this early post-operative hypotony [28].

2. *Elevated intraocular pressure*: Early post-operative high IOP is common in non-valved device. The tube occlusion suture by vicryl dissolves within 4–6 weeks and IOP tends to be in normal range by this period. So high IOP during this 4–6 weeks time can be treated by anti-glaucoma medications. Some surgeons combine a trabeculectomy without mitomycin C with the drainage device to prevent this post-operative high IOP [29].

3. *Tube migration, erosion and extrusion*: Tube migration is not uncommon. The tube may migrate both posteriorly or anteriorly. In the case of tube shortening, tube extender can be used to increase its size. The tube may migrate anteriorly due to dislocation of the external plate. In that case, it may require repositioning of the plate and tube and securing it to the sclera with additional 9-0 nylon sutures [30]. Tube exposure and erosion may require a new donor scleral graft to cover the tube.

4. *Endophthalmitis*: It has been seen in the Tube versus Trabeculectomy (TVT) study that endophthalmitis is less common in the tube group than trabeculectomy group [30].

   In most cases, tube exposure is the cause of infection. Surgical cleaning and revision are required and usually, the donor scleral graft is changed with a new one.

   If infection or endophthalmitis occurs within 1–2 weeks post-operatively, the implant should be removed and appropriate treatment of endophthalmitis should be done.

5. *Ocular motility disturbance:* Ocular motility disturbances, diplopia or strabismus are common in larger sized plates and if implanted in the superonasal quadrant. Here the plate is more anteriorly placed and can interrupt the function of extraocular muscles.

6. *Retinal complications*: If post-operative hypotony occurs for a prolonged time, it may cause suprachoroidal effusions, suprachoroidal haemorrhage, vitreous haemorrhage or retinal detachment [28]. Hypotony should be treated promptly to prevent retinal complications.

References

1. Quigley HA, Broman T. The number of people with glaucoma worldwide in 2010 and 2020. Br J Ophthalmol. 2006;90:262–7.
2. Foster PJ, Buhrman R, Quigley HA, Jhonson GJ. The definition and classification of glaucoma in prevalence surveys. Br J Ophthalmol. 2002 Feb;86(2):238–42.
3. Cairns JE. Trabeculectomy. Preliminary report of a new method. Am J Ophthalmol. 1968;66:673.
4. Varma D, Baylis O, Wride N, et al. Viscogonioplasty: an effective procedure for lowering intraocular pressure in primary angle closure glaucoma.May 2007; Eye. 21(4):472–5. https://doi.org/10.1038/sj.eye.6702224.PubMed.
5. Mermoud A, Schnyder CC, Sickenberg M, Chiou AG, Hediguer SE, Faggioni R. Comparison of deep sclerectomy with collagen implant and trabeculectomy in open-angle glaucoma. J Cataract Refract Surg. 1999;25:323–31.
6. Aung T, Tow SL, Yap EY, Chan SP, Seah SK. Trabeculectomy for acute primary angle closure. Ophthalmology. 2000;107:1298–302.
7. Brincker P, Kessing SV. Limbus-based versus fornix-based conjunctival flap in glaucoma filtering surgery. Acta Ophthalmol. 1992;70:641–4.
8. Khan AM, Jilani FA. Comparative results of limbal based versus fornix based conjunctival flaps for trabeculectomy. Indian J Ophthalmol. 1992;40:41–3.
9. Samsuddin APD, Eames IPD, Brocchini SPD, Khaw Peng Tee PD. The influence of scleral flap thickness, shape, and structures on intraocular pressure (IOP) and aqueous humour flow direction in a trabeculectomy model. J Glaucoma. 2016;25(7):704–12.
10. Suzuki R. Trabeculectomy with a Kelly Descemet membrane punch. Ophthalmologica. 1997;211(2):93–4.
11. Wand M. Intraoperative intracameral viscoelastic agent in the prevention of postfiltration flat anterior chamber. J Glaucoma. 1994;3(2):101–5.
12. de Barros DSM, Da Silva RS, Siam GA, Gheith ME, Nunes CM, Lankaranian D, Tittler EH, Myers JS, Spaeth GL. Should an iridectomy be routinely performed as a part of trabeculectomy? Two surgeons' clinical experience. Eye. 2009;23:362–7.

13. Faggioni R. Trabeculectomy with conjunctival flap in the fornix: 12 months' follow-up. Klin Monatsbl Augenheilkd. 1983;182(5):385–6.
14. Krebs DB, Liebmann JM, Ritch R, et al. Late infectious endophthalmitis from exposed glaucoma setons. Arch Ophthalmol. 1992;110(2):174–5.
15. Ball SF, Herrington RG. Long-term retention of chromic occlusion suture in glaucoma seton tubes. Arch Ophthalmol. 1993;111(2):169.
16. Lai JSM, Tham CCY, Lam DSC. Incisional surgery for angle closure glaucoma. J Semin Ophthalmol. 2002;2:92–9.
17. Tham CCY, Kwong YYY, Lai JSM, Lam DSC, Ritch R. Surgical management of chronic angle-closure glaucoma. J Exp Rev Ophthalmol. 2007;2(2): 185–90.
18. Rulli E, Biagioli E, Riva I, Gambirasio G, De Simone I, Floriani I, Quaranta L. Efficacy and safety of trabeculectomy vs nonpenetrating surgical procedures a systematic review and meta-analysis. JAMA Ophthalmol. 2013;131(12):1573–82.
19. O'Brart DPS, Shiew M, Edmunds B. A randomised, prospective study comparing trabeculectomy with viscocanalostomy with adjunctive antimetabolite usage for the management of open angle glaucoma uncontrolled by medical therapy. Br J Ophthalmol. 2004 Aug;88(8):1012–7.
20. Netland PA. Nonpenetrating glaucoma surgery. Ophthalmology. 2001;108:416–21.
21. Singh P, Kuldeep K, Tyagi M, Sharma PD, Kumar Y. Glaucoma drainage devices. JCOR. 2013;1(2):77–82.
22. Molteno AC. New implant for draining in glaucoma. Br J Ophthalmol. 1969;53:609.
23. Every SG, Molteno ACB, Bevin TH, et al. Long-term results of Molteno implant insertion in cases of Neovascular Glaucoma. Arch Ophthalmol. 2006;124(3):355–60.
24. Budenz DL, Barton K, Feuer WJ, et al. Treatment outcomes in the Ahmed Baerveldt comparison study after one year of follow-up. Ophthalmology. 2011;118:443–52.
25. Rathi SG, Seth NG, Kaur S, et al. A prospective randomized controlled study of Aurolab aqueous drainage implant versus Ahmed glaucoma valve in refractory glaucoma: a pilot study. Indian J Ophthalmol. 2018;66:1580–5.
26. Wilson MR, Mendis U, Paliwal A, et al. Long-term follow-up of primary glaucoma surgery with Ahmed glaucoma valve implant versus trabeculectomy. Am J Ophthalmol. 2003;136:464–70.
27. Fellenbaum PS, Almeida AR, Minckler DS, Sidoti PA. Krupin disk implantation for complicated glaucomas. Ophthalmology. 1994;101(7):1178–82.
28. Giovingo MC. Complications of Glaucoma drainage device surgery: a review. Semin Ophthalmol. 2014;29(5–6):397–402.
29. Kook MS, Yoon J, Kim J, Lee MS. Clinical results of Ahmed glaucoma valve implantation in refractory glaucoma with adjunctive mitomycin C. Ophthalmic Surg Lasers. 2000;31:100–6.
30. Gedde SJ, Schiffman JC, Feuer WJ, et al. Treatment outcomes in the tube versus trabeculectomy (TVT) study after five years of follow-up. Am J Ophthalmol. 2012;153:789–803.

Cyclodestructive Procedures

Isabel S. W. Lai, Claire Chow,
and Clement C. Y. Tham

Abstract

Cyclodestructive procedures target the aqueous pathway at the inflow level and provide an alternative treatment to filtering surgeries. The techniques have evolved over the last century and cyclophotocoagulation has emerged as the mainstay of cyclodestructive therapy. The transcleral diode cyclophotocoagulation is widely used but the potential complications of pain, hyphema, vision loss, hypotony, and phthisis have limited its use to mostly refractory glaucoma patients with poor visual potential.

However, with the recent advances of the newer cyclodestructive techniques, including micropulse transcleral cyclophotocoagulation (MP-TSCPC) and endoscopic cyclophotocoagulation (ECP), there is an emerging paradigm shift to offer these as surgical options in eyes with less severe glaucoma and good visual potential.

Keywords

Cyclodestructive procedures
Cyclophotocoagulation · Laser diode
Endoscopic · Transcleral · Ciliary body
Micropulse

I. S. W. Lai (✉) · C. Chow · C. C. Y. Tham
Department of Ophthalmology and Visual Sciences,
The Chinese University of Hong Kong, Hong Kong
Eye Hospital, Hong Kong, SAR, China

11.1 Introduction

Elevated intraocular pressure (IOP) is the most important modifiable risk factor for glaucoma. To lower the IOP, the aqueous pathway can be targeted at either the inflow or outflow level. Whereas filtering surgeries aim to lower the IOP by improving the aqueous outflow, cyclodestructive procedures aim to reduce aqueous humor production. This is achieved through damage to the secretory epithelium of the ciliary processes. Reduction of aqueous secretion decreases IOP and slows the progression of glaucoma [1].

The first use of cyclodestructive procedures to lower IOP date back to the early twentieth century, using a variety of methods including surgical excision, [2] diathermy, [3, 4] cryotherapy, ultrasound, microwave, and laser light of various wavelengths. Historically, cyclodestruction has been reserved for refractory glaucoma patients with poor visual potential, due to the associated severe complications with earlier technologies, including pain, hyphema, severe inflammation, visual loss, hypotony, and phthisis. However, with the recent advances of the newer cyclodestructive techniques, including micropulse transcleral cyclophotocoagulation (MP-TSCPC) and endoscopic cyclophotocoagulation (ECP), there is an emerging paradigm shift to offer these as surgical options in eyes with less severe glaucoma and good visual potential.

11.2   Cyclophotocoagulation (CPC)

Due to the complications associated with the older methods of cyclodestructive techniques, including cyclodiathermy and cyclocryotherapy, laser cyclophotocoagulation (CPC) has emerged as the mainstay of cyclodestructive therapy during the last five decades. CPC refers to the use of laser energy for the destruction of ciliary epithelial tissue. The mechanism of action is thought to be multifactorial, largely through aqueous suppression caused by coagulative necrosis of the secretory ciliary epithelium following the absorption of laser energy by the pigmented ciliary epithelium [5]. Supplementary mechanisms are tissue ischemia due to vascular damage from the dissipated laser energy from the ciliary epithelium to nearby vessels in the ciliary processes, and tissue disruption with micro-explosions often audible as "pop" sounds.

Although it is widely accepted that the effects of cyclodestructive procedures are mainly mediated through the inflow, there is evidence indicating that transscleral CPC may also increase ciliary body and scleral permeability to aqueous humor, thereby promoting the uveoscleral outflow pathway [6, 7].

CPC can be delivered in various ways namely: (1) Transscleral CPC (TSCPC); (2) Endoscopic CPC (ECP); and (3) Transpupillary CPC (TPCPC).

11.3   Transscleral Cyclophotocoagulation (TSCPC)

TSCPC can be performed with the contact and noncontact Neodymium: Yttrium-Aluminum-Garnet (Nd:YAG) laser (1064 nm), or the semiconductor diode laser (810 nm). Historically, Smith and Stein first proposed the use of ruby and Nd:YAG lasers for transscleral CPC in 1969 [8]. Then Beckman et al. reported the first use of ruby laser for transscleral CPC in 1972, [9] which was followed by the more effective Nd:YAG laser the following year [10]. In 1992, Hennis

and Stewart introduced the use of diode laser for transscleral CPC [11]. Of the different types of lasers, diode laser is the most widely used owing to its lower cost, efficiency, and portability [12]. Following all types of TSCPC, topical steroids and cycloplegic agents or systemic pain relief medications are administered.

11.4   Nd-YAG Cyclophotocoagulation

The use of Nd:YAG laser for transscleral ciliary body ablation has greater scleral penetration than using argon and diode, both of which have shorter wavelengths. Both contact and noncontact methods of laser delivery are conducted under peribulbar or retrobulbar anesthesia.

Noncontact Nd:YAG laser CPC (for example, Microruptor II or continuous wave Microruptor III from H.S. Meridian Inc.) is performed at the slit lamp and uses thermal pulsed mode of 20 ms duration with power titrated from 5 up to 9 Joules per application [12, 13]. It contains a helium-neon aiming beam that focuses on the conjunctiva, while the focus of the treating laser beam is offset at 3.6 mm into the eye. An eyelid speculum can be used to retract the lids during the procedure, or a contact lens can be placed, which has markings parallel to the limbus to guide laser application. Laser beam is applied to the sclera at 1.5 mm posterior to the surgical limbus superiorly and inferiorly, and 1 mm posterior to the surgical limbus nasally and temporally [12]. Approximately 30–40 laser spots are applied evenly over 360 degrees, [12] avoiding 3 and 9 o'clock positions to avoid damage to the long posterior ciliary nerves. Reduced treatment to 180 degrees may be considered in cases with an increased risk of hypotony [13].

Contact Nd:YAG laser CPC (Microruptor III, H.S. Meridian Inc.) is performed with the patient in supine position. A lid speculum is used to retract eyelids. The laser probe is oriented perpendicular to the sclera and the anterior edge of the sapphire probe connected to a fiberoptic handpiece is positioned at 0.5–1.0 mm posterior to the limbus. Approximately 16–40 laser spots are applied over 360 degrees, again sparing 3 and 9 o'clock positions, and power is titrated from 4 to 7 Watts for a duration of 0.5–0.7 s [12]. Patients may be retreated if there is inadequate intraocular pressure lowering at 1–4 weeks after the initial treatment, but retreatment uses half the number of initial laser applications to reduce the risk of hypotony and phthisis [14].

11.5 Semiconductor Diode Laser Cyclophotocoagulation

The semiconductor diode laser system (for example, Iridex IQ810 laser system, Fig. 11.1) consists of a G-probe (Fig. 11.2) which has a fiberoptic pit that is designed to direct the laser beam over the ciliary processes when it is placed at 1.2 mm from the corneoscleral limbus. The laser is applied with the patient in a supine position with

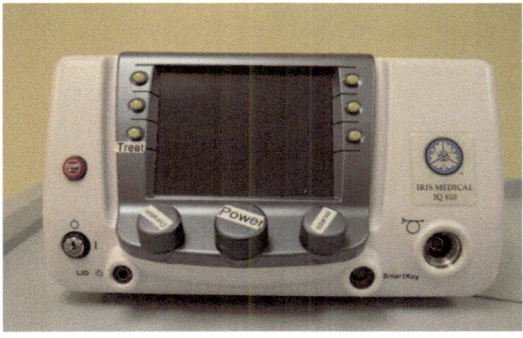

Fig. 11.1 The Iridex IQ 810 laser system used for diode laser cyclophotocoagulation

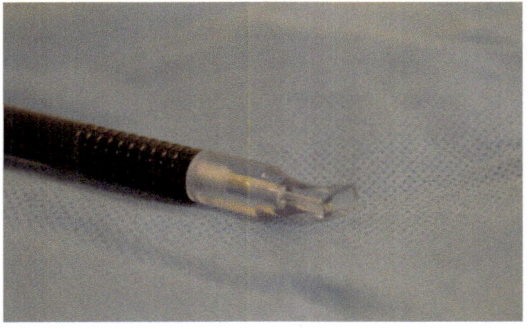

Fig. 11.2 The G-probe in diode laser cyclophotocoagulation (Iridex IQ810 laser system)

eyelid speculum insertion and under peribulbar or retrobulbar anesthesia. Laser settings typically start at an energy level of 1750 mW and are titrated in increments of 250 mW to a maximum of 2500 mW at a duration of 2000 msec. Power is titrated against an audible "pop" sound which represents the micro-explosion of the ciliary body and signifies the need to reduce the power [15]. Approximately 16–20 laser spots can be applied over 360 degrees, also avoiding the 3 and 9 o'clock positions.

11.6 Micropulse Transscleral Cyclophotocoagulation (MPCPC)

The micropulse diode laser system (Iridex Cyclo G6 glaucoma laser system, Fig. 11.3) is a novel method that delivers thermal energy in alternating "on" and "off" cycle mode. The advantage of this system is that it minimizes collateral damage when compared to older forms of transscleral cyclophotocoagulation. Short (microsecond) bursts of laser energy are delivered during the repetitive "on" cycles, which are absorbed by pigmented tissues of the ciliary processes and cause coagulative necrosis [16]. However, nonpigmented surrounding tissues are spared damage because the shorter bursts of laser energy do not allow these tissues to accumulate enough energy per unit time to meet the critical energy threshold needed for photocoagulation to take place. This is also assisted by the "off" cycles

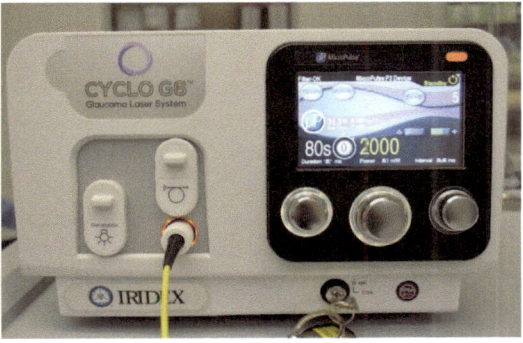

Fig. 11.3 The Iridex Cyclo G6 Micropulse laser system

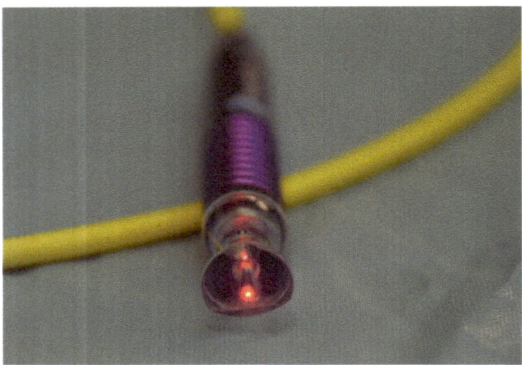

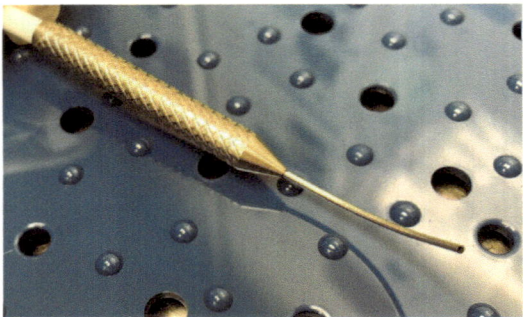

Fig. 11.5 Twenty-gage laser probe for endoscopic cyclophotocoagulation

Fig. 11.4 The laser probe used in the Iridex MicroPulse laser system has a specialized small groove that is to be aligned circumferential to the limbus during laser application

which help to dissipate energy between laser pulses. MPCPC is performed with the patient in supine position with the use of an eyelid speculum and under peribulbar or retrobulbar anesthesia. The design of the laser probe is different from the diode laser cyclophotocoagulation system in that it contains a groove that has to be aligned circumferential to the limbus during operation to help direct laser energy over the ciliary body (Fig. 11.4). Laser is applied at a power of 2000 mW using a duty cycle (the percentage of time that laser energy is delivered) of 31.33%, which consists of a micropulse "on" time of 0.5 ms and "off" time of 1.1 ms. [16] A total time of 100–240 s of treatment is conducted over 360 degrees, avoiding 3 and 9 o'clock positions [12].

11.7 Endoscopic Cyclophotocoagulation

Endoscopic Cyclophotocoagulation (ECP) is a cyclodestructive procedure in which the ciliary processes are photocoagulated under direct endoscopic visual guidance. It was first described by Uram in 1992 for IOP reduction in neovascular glaucoma [17]. Since then, ECP has gained popularity as a surgical option to treat glaucoma patients with moderate disease, especially in combination with phacoemulsification. Since the ciliary processes are directly visualized, they can

be treated precisely with diode laser energy, minimizing collateral damage. Hence the problems of pain, inflammation, hypotony, visual loss, and phthisis associated with transscleral cyclophotocoagulation are theoretically reduced and it can be used in eyes with excellent visual potential.

The laser endoscope for ECP has four components: a diode laser emitting pulsed continuous wave energy at 810 nm wavelength; a 175 W xenon light source; a helium-neon laser aiming beam, and a video camera for imaging and recording. ECP is performed through an 18-gage (1.2-mm diameter probe with viewing angle of 110°) or 20-gage (0.88-mm diameter probe with viewing angle of 70°) probe inserted intraocularly (Fig. 11.5). All elements of the probe are transmitted via fiberoptic. It is connected to a portable unit consisting of a video monitor, video recorder, and a control panel (Fig. 11.6). The surgeon performs the procedure by viewing the video monitor, rather than looking through the operating microscope (Fig. 11.7).

ECP can be performed through a limbal approach or a *pars plana* approach. The limbal approach is most commonly used as it can be performed in phakic, pseudophakia, or aphakic eyes. An incision size of 1.5–2.0 mm is created through the clear cornea or scleral tunnel. Viscoelastic is injected under the iris and above the ciliary processes to maximize the distance in the ciliary sulcus. This can facilitate the visualization of the ciliary processes and minimize the risk of thermal burn to the adjacent iris and inadvertent damage to the lens leading to cataract formation in

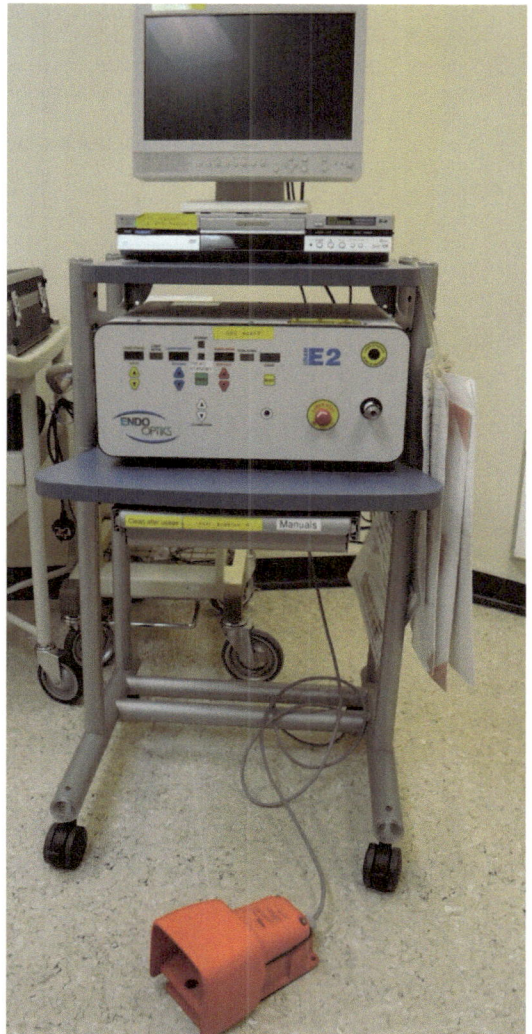

Fig. 11.6 The Endo Optiks E2 laser endoscopy system used for endoscopic cyclophotocoagulation is connected to a monitor to visualize direct laser application over the ciliary body via the endoscopic laser probe

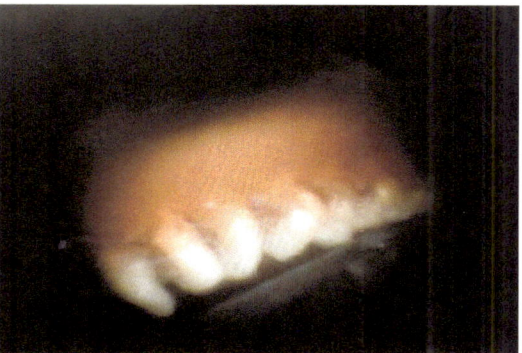

Fig. 11.7 Endoscopic view of photocoagulated ciliary processes. The whitening is a visible endpoint for photocoagulation

when excessive energy is used and should be avoided. Viscoelastic is then removed from the anterior chamber before wound closure.

The *pars plana* approach can be used for eyes with aphakia or pseudophakia, but the presence of the crystalline lens prohibits this option as the shaft of the endoscope may cause damage to the lens. After removal of the anterior vitreous, the laser endoscope is introduced through the *pars plana* 3.5 mm posterior to the limbus, and the ciliary processes are photocoagulated under endoscopic visualization.

11.8 Transpupillary Cyclophotocoagulation (TPCPC)

TPCPC employs the transmission of argon laser (488 nm) through the pupil to photocoagulate the visible ciliary processes. Its usage is limited to eyes in which there is clear visualization of a number of ciliary processes on gonioscopy, such as patients with aniridia, broad iridectomy, or extensive peripheral anterior synechiae causing anterior iris displacement. Typical settings are 700–740 mW of argon laser energy, 125 um spot size, and 0.3–0.5 s of pulse duration. A Goldmann gonioscopy lens can be used for the procedure.

phakic eyes. The typical laser energy setting for ECP is 200 mW and it is titrated until there are visible whitening and shrinkage of the ciliary processes. The entire ciliary process should be treated, from top to bottom. Typically, 180–360 degrees are treated with one or two corneal incisions. A pop sound or bubble formation is seen

11.9 Postoperative Management

After the procedure, patients may have their treated eye patched with combination topical ointment of dexamethasone, neomycin, and polymyxin B sulfates. They are prescribed topical steroid medication with or without topical antibiotics depending on infection risk and whether concomitant phacoemulsification was performed. Patients continue all topical and oral IOP-lowering medications at first. Patients return for follow up on postoperative day one to review the IOP and look for any procedure-related side effects. They return at postoperative 1 week and depending on the IOP, their usual IOP-lowering medications are slowly tapered or continued if insufficient IOP-lowering effect is seen. Topical steroids are gradually tapered off according to the degree of intraocular inflammation found on follow up visits and is usually prescribed for a duration of 4 weeks or more.

11.10 Complications

Traditionally, TSCPC was used as a last resort treatment for functional eyes with refractory glaucoma because of its high rate of complications [12]. It was also considered for use in eyes with poor visual prognosis. Known complications include pain, inflammation, hyphema, IOP fluctuations and hypotony, conjunctival burns, visual loss, cystoid macular edema, retinal detachment, and phthisis [18, 19]. The magnitude of energy used correlates with the risk of complications [18]. On the other hand, ECP has been found to have relatively lower rates of complication and is therefore frequently performed together with cataract surgery [18].

References

1. Lee DA, Higginbotham EJ. Glaucoma and its treatment: a review. Am J Health Syst Pharm: AJHP: Official Journal of the American Society of Health-System Pharmacists. 2005;62(7):691–9.
2. Verhoeff F. Cyclectomy: a new operation for glaucoma. Arch Ophthalmol. 1924;53:228–9.
3. Dunphy EB, Albaugh CH. Cyclodiathermy: an operation for the treatment of Glaucoma. Trans Am Ophthalmol Soc. 1941;39:193–213.
4. Shahan W, Post L. Thermophore studies in glaucoma. Am J Ophthalmol. 1921;4:109–18.
5. Ferry AP, King MH, Richards DW. Histopathologic observations on human eyes following neodymium: YAG laser cyclophotocoagulation for glaucoma. Trans Am Ophthalmol Soc 1995;93:315–331; discussion 32–6.
6. Liu GJ, Mizukawa A, Okisaka S. Mechanism of intra-ocular pressure decrease after contact transscleral continuous-wave Nd:YAG laser cyclophotocoagulation. Ophthalmic Res. 1994;26(2):65–79.
7. Schubert HD, Agarwala A, Arbizo V. Changes in aqueous outflow after in vitro neodymium: yttrium aluminum garnet laser cyclophotocoagulation. Invest Ophthalmol Vis Sci. 1990;31(9):1834–8.
8. Smith RS, Stein MN. Ocular hazards of transscleral laser radiation: II Intraocular injury produced by ruby and neodymium lasers. Am J Ophthalmol. 1969;67:100–10.
9. Beckman H, Kinoshita A, Rota A, Sugar H. Transscleral ruby laser irradiation of the ciliary body in the treatment of intractable glaucoma. Trans Am Acad Ophthalmol Otolaryngol. 1972;76:423–36.
10. Beckman H, Sugar HS. Neodymium laser cyclocoagulation. Arch Ophthalmol. 1973;90:27–8.
11. Hennis HL, Stewart WC. Semiconductor diode laser transscleral cyclophotocoagulation in patients with glaucoma. Am J Ophthalmol. 1992;113:81–5.
12. Ndulue JK, Rahmatnejad K, Sanvicente C, Wizoc SS, Moster MR. Evolution of cyclophotocoagulation. J Ophthalmic Vis Res. 2018;13:55–61.
13. Pastor SA, Singh K, Lee DA, Juzych MS, Lin SC, Netland PA, Nguyen NTA. Cyclophotocoagulation – a report by the American Academy of ophthalmology. Ophthalmology. 2001;108:2130–8.
14. Schuman JS, Bellows AR, Shingleton BJ, Latina MA, Allingham RR, Belcher CD, et al. Contact transscleral Nd: YAG laser cyclophotocoagulation. Midterm results. Ophthalmology. 1992;99:1089–95.
15. Schubert HD. The influence of exposure duration in transscleral Nd: YAG laser cyclophotocoagulation. Am J Ophthalmol. 1993;115:684.
16. Kuchar S, Moster MR, Reamer CB, Waisbourd M. Treatment outcomes of micropulse transscleral cyclophotocoagulation in advanced glaucoma. Lasers Med Sci. 2016;31:393.
17. Uram M. Ophthalmic laser microendoscope ciliary process ablation in the management of neovascular glaucoma. Ophthalmology. 1992;99(12):1823–8.
18. Ishida K. Update on results and complications of cyclophotocoagulation. Curr Opin Ophthalmol. 2013;24(2):102–10.
19. Kahook MY, Noecker RJ. Transscleral cyclophotocoagulation. Glaucoma Today. 2007 July/August:21–5.

Trabecular, Canal and Suprachoroidal Surgery in Primary Angle Closure

12

Paul R. Healey

Abstract

Angle surgery has always been the basis of the surgical management of angle closure and angle closure glaucoma. After iridectomy, cyclodialysis was the most effective surgery at the beginning of the twentieth century and by the 1930s, trabecular surgery in the form of goniotomy was popularised for open-angle disease. These operations have been rediscovered in the twenty-first century, forming the cornerstone of the MIGS procedures. Little modern evidence exists as to their utility in angle closure disease but what little there is suggests they may have a role once pupil block, lens crowding and synechial mechanisms have been controlled.

Keywords

Angle Closure · Glaucoma · MIGS
Goniotomy · Stent · Surgery · Suprachoroidal
Trabecular · Schlemm

This chapter will examine currently available surgical operations and devices for glaucoma which involve the trabecular/canal or suprachoroidal outflow pathways, the potentials and pitfalls of these procedures in the management of Primary Angle Closure and the current evidence of their safety and effectiveness. Goniosynechialysis is covered in a separate chapter.

12.1 The Development of Trabecular, Canal and Suprachoroidal Surgery

All currently available trabecular and suprachoroidal surgical devices approved for the treatment of glaucoma are approved for open-angle glaucoma and not angle closure glaucoma. This does not mean that angle and suprachoroidal surgeries are ineffective in primary angle closure. Indeed the first successful operation to lower intraocular pressure in glaucoma was angle surgery. It was pioneered by Albrecht von Graefe in the 1850s and was called Iridectomy. The technique

P. R. Healey (✉)
Sydney Medical School, University of Sydney, Sydney, Australia

University of Sydney, Centre for Vision Research, Westmead Millennium Institute and Save Sight Institute, Sydney, Australia

Sydney Eye Hospital, Sydney, Australia

Westmead Hospital, Westmead, NSW, Australia

Eye Associates, Sydney, NSW, Australia
e-mail: Paul.Healey@Sydney.edu.au

© Springer Nature Singapore Pte Ltd. 2021
C. C. Y. Tham (ed.), *Primary Angle Closure Glaucoma (PACG)*,
https://doi.org/10.1007/978-981-15-8120-5_12

involved tearing or cutting out a fairly large area of the root of the iris and while used in many types of glaucoma, was most effective in the congestive types which included most angle closure disease associated with a very elevated intraocular pressure [1]. At the time, the mechanism of action was unknown. Gonioscopy would not be invented for another half-century. But with hindsight and modern understanding of the glaucomas which present with very elevated intraocular pressure, the mechanism was most probably threefold: breaking of pupil block, removal of irido-trabecular contact, and in some cases at least, creation of a cyclodialysis cleft.

The idea of lowering the pressure in glaucoma by creating a communication between the anterior chamber and the suprachoroidal space started with a paper by Ernest Fuchs in 1900, describing hypotony with a flat anterior chamber and choroidal effusion following cataract extraction with iridectomy, where choroidal tissue was also removed [2]. In 1905, Leopold Heine described an operation to intentionally create a to lower intraocular pressure also in congestive glaucoma. He called this the Cyclodialysis [3].

The third key intraocular operation to lower pressure in glaucoma involved incision through or removal of some part of the trabecular meshwork and the inner wall of the canal of Schlemm. The idea that an incision of the iridocorneal angle could lower intraocular pressure was promoted by Carlos de Vincentiis [4] in the 1890s. However, without any way to view the angle, the results were unpredictable and generally disappointing.

With the development of gonioscopy in the early 1900s, primarily by Alexios Trantas [5, 6], and the development of the direct gonioscopy lens by Leonhard Koeppe [7], it became possible for surgeons to actually see what they were doing in the angle. Otto Barkan initially performed an incision of the angle in the manner described by de Vincentiis. Concerned by the risks of incising iris root or cornea unseen, he brought together a binocular microscope, carbon-arc slit lamp illumination system and a modified Koeppe lens allowing incision through the trabecular meshwork under direct magnified stereoscopic vision [8]. He performed this operation in primary and secondary chronic 'non-congestive' glaucomas (importantly noting his preference to define the glaucoma gonioscopically as having an open or narrow angle), in adults and reported excellent results in the open-angle type. While he initially described this accurately as 'intraocular microsurgery', he later coined the term 'goniotomy' for the procedure. He did not perform the procedure in the presence of peripheral anterior synechiae and thought it most probably was a contraindication. Over the next few years, it became apparent that the procedure was unreliable in adult glaucoma but highly effective in congenital glaucoma [9].

Trabeculotomy was an ab externo procedure attempting to achieve a similar outcome to goniotomy. It was described in 1960 by Redmond Smith using a suture [10] and Hermann Burian using a specially manufactured 'trabeculotome' [11]. Theoretically, the difference between goniotomy and trabeculotomy was that the latter incised the inner wall of Schlemm's canal as well as the trabecular meshwork, whereas the former only incised the trabecular meshwork. Practically, the latter provided a little more certainty of anatomy (if the canal could be found) and allowed surgery in an eye with a cloudy cornea, at the cost of traumatising the conjunctiva and sclera. Like goniotomy, it was not reliable in adults, but found a place in the treatment of congenital glaucoma. Neither of these operations removed tissue. That operation was called a 'trabeculectomy' and reported by J Cairns in 1968 as a more effective way to ensure patency of the trabeculotomy [12]!

The beginning of the twenty-first century saw a resurgence in intraocular microsurgery for glaucoma. All the previously abandoned operations were reinvestigated with an interest in the relatively low symptoms and side effects compared with trabeculectomy but the challenge of changing them to overcome early failure.

For goniotomy, the perceived problem was as Cairns postulated when he described trabeculectomy [12], that trabecular tissue had to be completely removed to prevent tissue around the incision from blocking the stoma. This was achieved with the Trabectome device (NeoMedix

Corporation in Tustin, CA, USA) using diathermy [13] and the Kahook Dual blade (New World Medical, Rancho Cucamonga, CA, USA) [14] by excising a strip of trabecular meshwork and inner wall of Schlemm's canal.

A novel prosthetic alternative to these excisional techniques was to implant a microstent through the trabecular meshwork and inner canal wall. Glaukos Corporation (San Clemente, CA, USA) developed two such stents, the iStent [15] and subsequently, the iStent Inject [16]. Ivantis Corporation (Irvine, CA, USA) developed the Hydrus microstent which combined transtrabecular micro-bypass with stenting of 3 clock hours of the canal [17].

For cyclodialysis, the perceived problem was two-fold; the tendency for initial marked hypotony due to too much flow, and subsequently marked failure from scarring closure of the cleft. The solution was a prosthesis which aimed to simultaneously control flow and prevent cleft closure. The Cypass [18] (Alcon, Fort Worth, TX, USA) and iStent Supra [19] (Glaukos, San Clemente, CA, USA) are both small rigid tubes inserted into a cyclodialysis cleft with a fixed diameter to control flow. The iStent supra additionally has a coating of Heparin. In 2018, the Cypass stent was withdrawn from sale over concerns about a 5-year loss of corneal endothelial cells in some eyes. The iStent Supra is yet to be approved for use.

The last set of procedures to lower intraocular pressure focussed on the canal of Schlemm itself. A report by Robert Stegman in 1999 of combining a deep sclerectomy with the injection of viscoelastic into the canal of Schlemm (called a viscocanalostomy) [20] generated interest in the idea of dilating the canal with viscoelastic with or without a tensioned suture (called canaloplasty) [21]. These were all ab externo operations that were based on deep sclerectomy techniques, making it difficult to judge which part of the operation was responsible for outcomes. More recently, an ab interno approach has been developed using a flexible microcatheter passed through a goniotomy to dilate and inject viscoelastic into the canal (ab interno canaloplasty or AbIC) [22].

12.2 The Role of Trabecular, Canal and Suprachoroidal Surgery in Primary Angle Closure

A clear theme evolving in this textbook is the role of irido-trabecular apposition and adhesion in the development of primary angle closure and the importance of removing it in the treatment of this condition. As delineated in other chapters, peripheral iridotomy and iridectomy are very effective in abolishing pupil block and lens extraction in facilitating the iris and other anterior uveal structures to move posteriorly. These actions are effective in removing irido-trabecular apposition. Where peripheral anterior synechiae exist, goniosynechialysis effectively removes most iris tissue leaving the internal face of the trabecular meshwork once again in contact with the aqueous.

The need for chapters on filtration surgery and cyclodestruction suggests that restoring conventional outflow structure does not always restore function. This is not surprising given the degree to which trabecular function can be impaired by pigment or pseudoexfoliation material. Given the primacy of irido-trabecular apposition in elevating intraocular pressure in angle closure, it is reasonable to expect that the increased outflow resistance would be found within the trabecular meshwork itself, rather than the canal of Schlemm, collector channels or other parts of the distal outflow pathway. This, as well as the somewhat higher complication rates for glaucoma filtering surgery, makes trabecular surgery appealing when the angle has already been opened by the methods outlined above. While one might think of this situation as residual 'open-angle' disease, the outcomes of trabecular surgery in this population may not be the same as in those whose angles have always been open and specific studies are required to evaluate whether this is the case.

Whilst cyclodialysis is a different drainage pathway to trabecular surgery, it requires access to the root of the iris which lies below the scleral spur. Thus at least a localised goniosynechialysis is required to implant a suprachoroidal stent. Whilst supraciliary effusions from drained aqueous may cause anterior rotation of the ciliary body, suprachoroidal drainage may nevertheless have fewer downsides than trabeculectomy in patients with small eyes and angle closure.

Canaloplasty would necessarily require an open angle as no amount of canal dilatation would increase the hydraulic conductivity of the iris. If, however, the mechanism of action of canaloplasty includes a form of micro-perforating trabeculotomy induced by the high pressure in the canal, there may be unexpected pressure lowering with this procedure in primary angle closure.

The question of whether the technology is useful when the angle has not been opened is more complex. Assuming the posterior pressure on the iris has been removed, the benefit of a stent of small cross-sectional area (be it trabecular or suprachoroidal) is that it only needs a small area of open angle to be inserted. Its limitation is that only a small amount of iris needs to come into contact with the stent to block it. In contrast, the excision of trabecular tissue necessarily requires more trabecular tissue to be accessible, although the optimal amount may not be able to be assumed from trials in open-angle glaucoma. Whilst a larger amount of iris would be required to block it, higher outflow would create a larger pressure gradient between anterior and posterior chambers, which may draw the iris into the newly made outflow pathway. It is clear, therefore, that clinical practice will need to be supported by clinical trial evidence.

12.3 Clinical Studies of Trabecular and Suprachoroidal Surgery in Primary Angle Closure

The literature of clinical studies of trabecular and suprachoroidal surgery in primary angle closure and primary angle closure glaucoma is sparse. Chansangpetch et al. [23] performed a retrospective review of 301 eyes of 241 consecutive patients with primary glaucoma who had undergone uncomplicated cataract surgery, some of whom also had iStent implantation at the time, at

a single centre in CA, USA. All eyes in the study either had angles open to at least Shaffer grade 2 for ≥180 degrees (open-angle group) or Shaffer grading of ≥1 for ≥180 degrees, which deepened to grade ≥2 after preoperative laser peripheral iridotomy but who still had intraocular pressure considered too high and/or requiring glaucoma medications. Whilst peripheral anterior synechiae were not considered exclusion criteria, when they were present in the nasal angle to a degree that concerned the investigators, the eye was excluded from the study. The reason why some eyes received iStent but others did was not reported. Of the 301 eyes, 93 with angle closure had cataract extraction and 87 with angle closure had cataract extraction and iStent. At 12 months after surgery, 43.7% of iStent group had intraocular pressures ≤18 mmHg without medication compared with 37.6% who had no iStent. Mean medication reduction was 1.54 in the iStent group compared with 0.74 in the cataract only group. The additional benefit of the iStent was not statistically significantly different between the angle closure and open-angle groups despite the fact that cataract extraction alone was more successful in bringing the unmedicated intraocular pressure to 18 mmHg or less in the angle closure group compared with either arm of the open-angle group.

A 12-month case series of iStent implantation at the time of lens extraction surgery has been reported by Hernstadt et al. [24] Subjects with newly diagnosed Primary Angle Closure (IOP >23 mmHg, posterior trabecular meshwork not visible on gonioscopy in primary position for at least 180 degrees) or Primary Angle Closure Glaucoma (above with glaucomatous optic neuropathy) who required at least one glaucoma medication were recruited prospectively at two tertiary referral centres in Singapore. Those agreeing to have lens phacoemulsification, intraocular lens and iStent had the opportunity to pay for a second iStent if they wished. Of the 31 patients enrolled, 37 eyes had surgery, of which 16 eyes had two iStents. Medicated intraocular pressure was reduced from 17.5 mmHg to 14.8 mmHg with an additional reduction of medications from 1.49 to 0.14 per eye. Ten eyes (27%) had occlusion of the iStent by the iris, of which occlusion was partial in five. This is a higher rate than the 4–18% reported in similar open-angle glaucoma cohorts [25]. Higher preoperative intraocular pressure and deeper anterior chamber were associated with increased risk of stent occlusion. The authors reasoned that angle closure patients with deeper anterior chambers were more likely to have non-pupil-block angle-crowding mechanisms such as plateau iris configuration or a prominent last iris roll, predisposing the stent to occlusion.

There has been one case series reporting outcomes of the iStent Inject in various types of glaucoma including angle closure [26]. All were in conjunction with cataract surgery and in all but two of 165 eyes, two stents were injected as per the manufacturer's recommendations. Only 11 eyes had appositional angle closure or were primary angle closure suspects and outcomes in this group were not separately reported. However, amongst reported complications, there was only one case of intermittent iris-stent touch with no sequelae at 12 months and no cases of stent occlusion.

In a review of the Trabectome Study Group database, a post-marketing surveillance database, Bussel analysed outcomes according to Shaffer angle grade in phakic patients and patients where the trabectome surgery was combined with cataract surgery [27]. Of 671 eyes, 91 were Shaffer grade 1 or 2; 8 grade 1 phakic eyes had trabectome surgery and a further 6 had trabectome surgery combined with cataract surgery. For grade 2, the numbers were 35 and 42, respectively. In those with Shaffer grading ≤2, trabectome surgery reduced intraocular pressure from 27.3 mmHg to 15.7 mmHg in phakic eyes and from 20.7 mmHg to 15.7 mmHg in the combined group at 1 year. Despite a 97% power to detect a difference of 3 mmHg between this group and 580 eyes with Shaffer grade > 2, no differences were found in any efficacy parameter, nor were differences in complications found based on angle width. Estimates were similar in the phakic and combined surgery groups, although failure (25% vs 7%) and the need for secondary surgery

(21% vs 3%) were much higher in the phakic group than the combined group, irrespective of angle width.

There is a single published case report of implantation of the Cypass suprachoroidal shunt in a 19-year-old patient with pre-existing secondary angle closure from diabetic neovascularisation, pars planar vitrectomy and an Ahmed glaucoma drainage device. After cataract extraction and focal goniosynechialysis, a Cypass stent was inserted nasally with good pressure control on medications reported at 6 months [28]. In 2017, Wong and Leung presented outcomes of 11 eyes of phakic patients with primary angle closure or primary angle closure glaucoma who received a single iStent Supra implanted into the suprachoroidal space [29]. At 3 months, intraocular pressure had fallen from 23 mmHg to 18.6 mmHg with the number of medications decreasing from 2.8 to 2.1. No intraoperative complications or post-operative stent occlusions were reported.

There are no published studies on any canal-based procedure in angle closure.

12.4 Conclusions

Trabecular, suprachoroidal and canal surgery together make up the intraocular glaucoma surgery often referred to as Minimally or Micro-Invasive Glaucoma Surgery. The only truly new procedure is the canaloplasty/viscocanalostomy, which is the least likely to be beneficial in angle closure and for which there is no data yet in the literature. Goniotomy and Cyclodialysis were already well established as procedures that sometimes lower intraocular pressure very well but frequently fail in the longer term. The creation of precise biocompatible intraocular stents to facilitate and control flow is novel and what little evidence that does exist suggests that they may serve a role in eyes that have already had pupil block and lens mechanisms removed. Their ability to lower intraocular pressure appears similar to open-angle glaucoma with the reservation that stent occlusion is more likely if the angle remains crowded. The full effect of this potential problem and the potential benefit of pilocarpine or local iridotomy has not been explored. At this stage, there is no reason for surgeons experienced in this form of surgery not to consider these technologies in the management of their angle closure and angle closure glaucoma patients.

References

1. von Graefe A. Ueber die Iridectomie bei Glaucom und uber den glaucomatosen Process. Archiv für Opthalmologie. 1857;3(2):456–555.
2. Fuchs E. Ablösung der Aderhaut nach Staaroperation. Graefes Arhiv für Ophthalmologie. 1900;51(2):199–224.
3. Heine L. Die Cyclodialyse, eine neue Glaukomoperation. Dtsch Med Wschr. 1905:824–6.
4. Vincentiis D. Sulla incisione dell'angolo irideo (contribuzione all cura del glaucoma). Ann Otamol (Pavia). 1891;22:540.
5. Trantas A. Moyens d'explorer par l'ophtalmoscope – et par translucidité – la partie antérieure du fond oculaire, le cercle ciliaire y compris. Arch Ophtalmol (Paris). 1900;20:314.
6. Trantas A. L'ophtalmoscopie de l'angle irido-corneen. Arch Ophtalmol (Paris). 1918;36:257–76.
7. Koeppe L. Ueber den derzeitigen Stand der Glaukomforschung an der Gullstrandschen Nernstpaltlampe sowie den weiteren Ausbau des Glaukoms. Fruhdiagnose vermittelst dieser Untersuchungsmethode. Z Augenheilk. 1918;40
8. Barkan O. A new operation for chronic Glaucoma: restoration of physiological function by opening Schlemm's canal under direct magnified vision. Am J Ophthalmol. 1936;19(11):951–66.
9. Barkan O. Surgery of congenital glaucoma; review of 196 eyes operated by goniotomy. Am J Ophthalmol. 1953;36(11):1523–34.
10. Smith R. A new technique for opening the canal of Schlemm. Preliminary report. Br J Ophthalmol. 1960;44:370–3.
11. Burian HM. A case of Marfan's syndrome with bilateral glaucoma. With description of a new type of operation for developmental glaucoma (trabeculotomy ab externo). Am J Ophthalmol. 1960;50:1187–92.
12. Cairns JE. Trabeculectomy. Preliminary report of a new method. Am J Ophthalmol. 1968;66(4):673–9.
13. Minckler D, Baerveldt G, Ramirez MA, Mosaed S, Wilson R, Shaarawy T, et al. Clinical results with the Trabectome, a novel surgical device for treatment of open-angle glaucoma. Trans Am Ophthalmol Soc. 2006;104:40–50.
14. Seibold LK, Soohoo JR, Ammar DA, Kahook MY. Preclinical investigation of ab interno trabeculectomy using a novel dual-blade device. Am J Ophthalmol. 2013;155(3):524–9e2.
15. Spiegel D, Wetzel W, Haffner DS, Hill RA. Initial clinical experience with the trabecular microbypass stent in patients with glaucoma. Adv Ther. 2007;24(1):161–70.
16. Bahler CK, Hann CR, Fjield T, Haffner D, Heitzmann H, Fautsch MP. Second-generation trabecular meshwork bypass stent (iStent inject) increases outflow facility in cultured human anterior segments. Am J Ophthalmol. 2012;153(6):1206–13.
17. Camras LJ, Yuan F, Fan S, Samuelson TW, Ahmed IK, Schieber AT, et al. A novel Schlemm's canal scaffold increases outflow facility in a human anterior segment perfusion model. Invest Ophthalmol Vis Sci. 2012;53(10):6115–21.
18. Hoeh H, Ahmed II, Grisanti S, Grisanti S, Grabner G, Nguyen QH, et al. Early postoperative safety and surgical outcomes after implantation of a suprachoroidal micro-stent for the treatment of open-angle glaucoma concomitant with cataract surgery. J Cataract Refract Surg. 2013;39(3):431–7.
19. Myers JS, Masood I, Hornbeak DM, Belda JI, Auffarth G, Junemann A, et al. Prospective evaluation of two iStent((R)) trabecular stents, one iStent supra((R)) Suprachoroidal stent, and postoperative prostaglandin in refractory Glaucoma: 4-year outcomes. Adv Ther. 2018;35(3):395–407.
20. Stegmann R, Pienaar A, Miller D. Viscocanalostomy for open-angle glaucoma in black African patients. J Cataract Refract Surg. 1999;25(3):316–22.
21. Lewis RA, von Wolff K, Tetz M, Korber N, Kearney JR, Shingleton B, et al. Canaloplasty: circumferential viscodilation and tensioning of Schlemm's canal using a flexible microcatheter for the treatment of open-angle glaucoma in adults: interim clinical study analysis. J Cataract Refract Surg. 2007;33(7):1217–26.
22. Gallardo MJ, Supnet RA, Ahmed IIK. Viscodilation of Schlemm's canal for the reduction of IOP via an ab-interno approach. Clin Ophthalmol. 2018;12:2149–55.
23. Chansangpetch S, Lau K, Perez CI, Nguyen N, Porco TC, Lin SC. Efficacy of cataract surgery with trabecular microbypass stent implantation in combined-mechanism angle closure Glaucoma patients. Am J Ophthalmol. 2018;195:191–8.
24. Hernstadt DJ, Cheng J, Htoon HM, Sangtam T, Thomas A, Sng CCA. Case series of combined iStent implantation and phacoemulsification in eyes with primary angle closure disease: one-year outcomes. Adv Ther. 2019;36(4):976–86.
25. Le K, Saheb H. iStent trabecular micro-bypass stent for open-angle glaucoma. Clin Ophthalmol. 2014;8:1937–45.

26. Clement CI, Howes F, Ioannidis AS, Shiu M, Manning D. One-year outcomes following implantation of second-generation trabecular micro-bypass stents in conjunction with cataract surgery for various types of glaucoma or ocular hypertension: multicenter, multi-surgeon study. Clin Ophthalmol. 2019;13:491–9.

27. Bussel II, Kaplowitz K, Schuman JS, Loewen NA, Trabectome Study G, Outcomes of ab interno trabeculectomy with the trabectome by degree of angle opening. Br J Ophthalmol. 2015;99(7):914–9.

28. Hopen ML, Patel S, Gallardo MJ. Cypass Supraciliary stent in eye with chronic angle closure and Postvitrectomy with silicone oil. J Glaucoma. 2018;27(10):e151–e3.

29. Wong O, Leung C. Safety and efficacy of suprachoroidal stent implantation in patients with primary angle closure/primary angle closure glaucoma. In: Association for research in vision and ophthalmology. Baltimore: IOVS; 2017.

Malignant Glaucoma and Choroidal Detachment after Drainage Surgery and Its Management

13

Tetsuya Yamamoto

Abstract

Appropriate management of early postoperative complications is key to the success of drainage surgery. Discussed here are diagnosis and management of two major early postoperative complications: malignant glaucoma and choroidal detachment, especially in eyes with primary angle-closure disease.

Keywords

Choroidal detachment · Malignant glaucoma Shallow anterior chamber · Trabeculectomy Drainage surgery · Primary angle closure

13.1 Introduction

Postoperative complications are common with surgery for primary angle-closure disease and may include malignant glaucoma and choroidal detachment following drainage surgery like trabeculectomy. This chapter discusses the diagnosis and management of these two major early postoperative complications.

T. Yamamoto (✉)
Professor Kazuo Iwata Memorial KAIJIN Glaucoma Center, Kaiya Eye Hospital, Hamamatsu, Japan
e-mail: tetsuya.yamamoto@kaiya.jp

13.2 Differential Diagnosis for Shallow Anterior Chamber after Drainage Surgery

The shallow anterior chamber is a common early postoperative complication following drainage or filtering surgery. The main causes include excessive filtration or overfiltration, choroidal detachment and hemorrhage, and malignant glaucoma. Table 13.1 presents the main considerations for the differential diagnosis of these causes. Excessive filtration exhibits a large filtering bleb and low intraocular pressure (IOP). Choroidal detachment exhibits a dome-like, non-hemorrhagic lesion in the peripheral retina with low IOP. Hemorrhagic choroidal detachment exhibits a dome-like, hemorrhagic lesion in the peripheral retina and elevated IOP. Malignant glaucoma features an extremely shallow anterior chamber and markedly elevated IOP.

13.3 Malignant Glaucoma

Malignant glaucoma is characterized by high IOP and an extremely shallow anterior chamber (Fig. 13.1). Additionally, the filtering bleb is usually flattened. In typical cases, IOP may be 50–60 mmHg, although it can remain within normal limits in some cases. The anterior chamber is absent or extremely shallow. Ultrasound biomi-

© Springer Nature Singapore Pte Ltd. 2021
C. C. Y. Tham (ed.), *Primary Angle Closure Glaucoma (PACG)*,
https://doi.org/10.1007/978-981-15-8120-5_13

Table 13.1 Differential diagnosis for shallow AC after trabeculectomy

Cause	Excessive filtration	Choroidal detachment	Choroidal hemorrhage	Malignant glaucoma
IOP	Low	Low	High	High-normal
AC depth	Shallow	Shallow-deep	Shallow-deep	Extremely shallow
Fundus	None	Dome-like	Dark-red dome-like	None
UBM	Huge bleb	Effusion	High intensity	Anteriorly located ciliary body

IOP intraocular pressure, *AC* anterior chamber, *UBM* ultrasound biomicroscopy

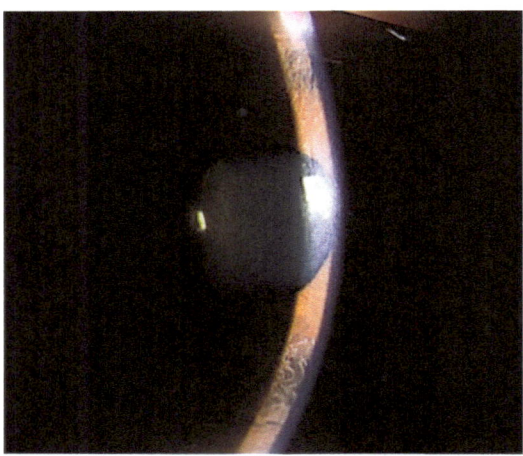

Fig. 13.1 Slit-lamp microscopy of malignant glaucoma. Anterior chamber is absent

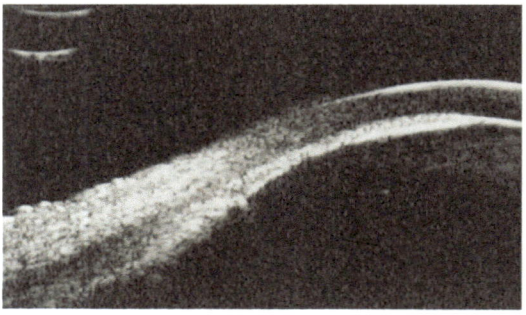

Fig. 13.2 Ultrasound biomicroscopic view of malignant glaucoma. Ciliary body is anteriorly located and flattened. Anterior chamber is absent

croscopy indicates an anteriorly located, flattened ciliary body in addition to a very shallow anterior chamber (Fig. 13.2), which is of extreme value for diagnosing this condition. B-mode echography may show no abnormality in the vitreous cavity, and ophthalmoscopy may likewise reveal no major abnormalities.

The term malignant glaucoma was coined to describe cases in which ordinary glaucoma treatment was non-effective and the prognosis was quite poor following peripheral iridectomy in eyes with acute angle-closure glaucoma. Although outcomes have been greatly improved, malignant glaucoma remains a serious condition that requires early diagnosis and prompt treatment upon diagnosis.

The incidence of malignant glaucoma following intraocular surgery in primary angle-closure glaucoma was reported to be 2–4% prior to 1951 [1]. It has decreased significantly in recent years, mainly due to improvements in diagnosis and treatment, and especially due to changes in surgical techniques for primary angle-closure disease. The incidence of primary angle-closure disease among all cases of malignant glaucoma remains high. He et al. [2] reported that all consecutive 30 cases of malignant glaucoma had had a diagnosis of acute or chronic angle-closure glaucoma or preclinical stage of acute angle-closure glaucoma. Balekudaru et al. [3] reported that 89.7% of their 58 cases were primary angle-closure glaucoma.

13.3.1 Pathogenesis of Malignant Glaucoma

Although the pathogenesis of malignant glaucoma remains uncertain, abnormal pooling of the aqueous humor in the vitreous cavity is hypothesized as the main mechanism. This hypothesis is supported by clinical findings such as anterior rotation of the ciliary body visualized via ultrasound biomicroscopy, and the efficacy of vitreous surgery. The basic mechanism of the intravitreous pooling is called ciliolenticular block or ciliary block. However, it may be more useful to view this condition as arising from several mechanisms, since malignant glaucoma develops based on several triggering pathologies, including the anatomical relationships among ciliary processes and the lens, lens zonules, and the anterior hyaloid membrane. Further, ciliary body edema, choroidal effusion, slackness of lens zonules, and inflammation all may play a role. Figure 13.3 summarizes some of the known mechanisms of malignant glaucoma in primary angle-closure disease.

13.3.2 Management of Malignant Glaucoma

Although it is generally preferable to initiate treatment medically, the surgical intervention must be performed without delay whenever indicated.

13.3.2.1 Medical Therapy

Cycloplegics cause the contraction of smooth muscle in the ciliary body, which retracts the lens zonules and helps break the ciliary block. Thus, they should be used intensively in both definite and suspected cases.

Hyperosmotic agents may also be useful. Their mechanism of action is to reduce the volume of the vitreous, thus lowering the pressure on the ciliary body. Likewise, there is a role for agents that reduce aqueous production. Among these, are carbonic anhydrase inhibitors, applied either topically or systemically, and beta-blockers. Topical steroids can also reduce intraocular inflammation and normalize the ciliary body.

13.3.2.2 Surgical Therapy

Surgical therapy for malignant glaucoma strives to create communication between the vitreous cavity and the anterior chamber, leading to a unicameral eye.

YAG laser posterior capsulotomy and/or anterior hyaloidotomy is effective in treating pseudophakia/aphakic malignant glaucoma. Laser photocoagulation of the ciliary processes may also be helpful.

When these abovementioned measures fail to break the ciliary block, vitrectomy is the treatment of choice. It is essential that the decision for surgical intervention is made promptly. Complete anterior vitrectomy is recommended, and lens extraction may also be indicated. Fortunately, recent studies have demonstrated a 90% rate of resolution of malignant glaucoma when vitreous surgery or modified vitrectomy combined with phacoemulsification is applied [2–4].

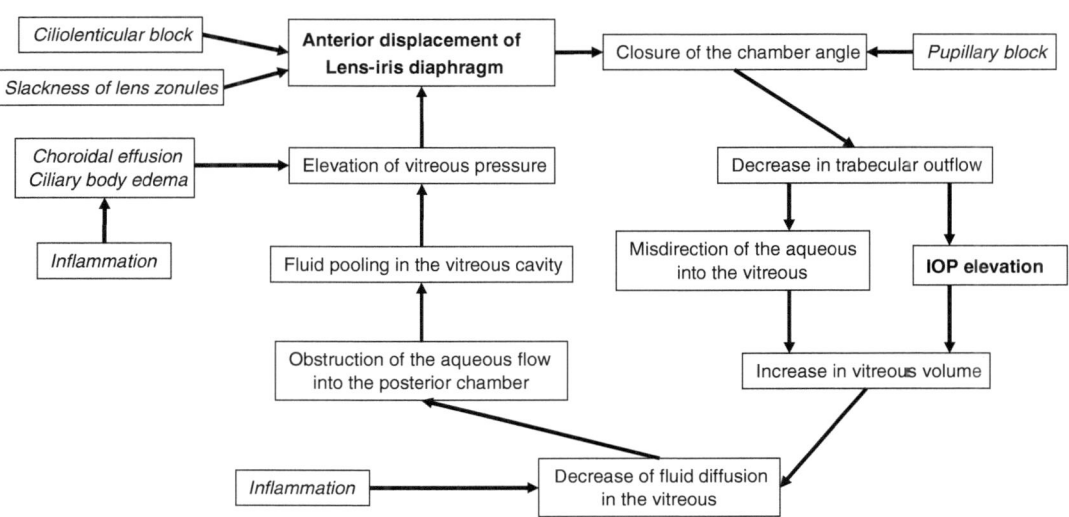

Fig. 13.3 Mechanism of malignant glaucoma in primary angle-closure disease

13.4 Choroidal Detachment

Choroidal detachment is recognized as a dome-like, non-hemorrhagic lesion at the peripheral retina (Fig. 13.4). It is usually accompanied by hypotony and a shallow anterior chamber. The IOP is usually 2–7 mmHg and choroidal detachment is rarely seen in eyes with an IOP ≥10 mmHg. In most cases, the anterior chamber depth is slightly to moderately shallow, but may also be normal. B-mode echography reveals intraocular hemi-circular, hollow lesion(s) in the vitreous cavity (Fig. 13.5). Ultrasound biomicroscopy reveals choroidal effusion in the most peripheral areas of the retina. The retina may be

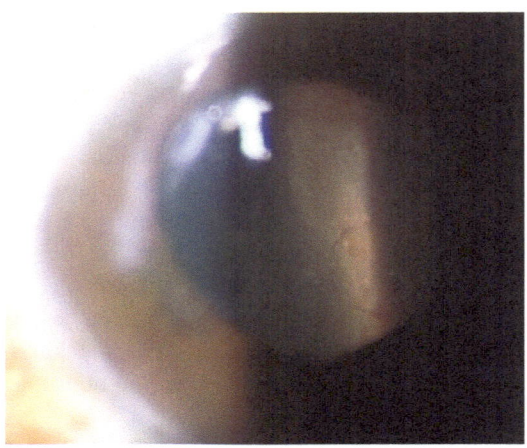

Fig. 13.6 Slit-lamp microscopy of choroidal detachment. Retina is partially visible

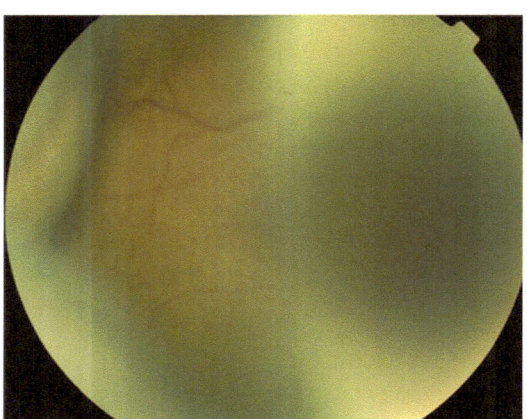

Fig. 13.4 Choroidal detachment. Recognized as a dome-like, non-hemorrhagic lesion

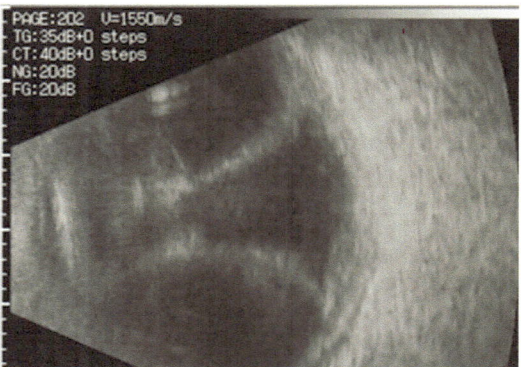

Fig. 13.5 B-mode echography of choroidal detachment, showing intraocular hemi-circular, hollow lesions in the vitreous

visible via slit-lamp microscopy in severe cases (Fig. 13.6). Primary angle closure is known to be a significant risk factor for the development of choroidal detachment [5]. The main strategy for managing choroidal detachment requires intervention in the hypotony and inflammation.

13.4.1 Pathogenesis of Choroidal Detachment

The pathogenesis of choroidal detachment is complicated, involving low IOP, inflammation, an abnormally high-pressure difference across the choroidal vessel, compression of the vortex vein, and other mechanisms yet to be identified [6].

Under normal conditions, suprachoroidal fluid, if present, drains out of the eye mainly via vortex veins; whereas, in eyes with low IOP, the force driving fluid drainage, which arises from the venous pressure differential within and without the eye, is significantly reduced due to lowered IOP. Hence, the fluid accumulates in the suprachoroidal space. This is understandable since uveoscleral outflow is reduced in eyes with extremely low IOP, whereas it is nearly constant at every IOP level except with markedly low IOP. Hypotony also causes choroidal detachment, which may reduce aqueous production leading to prolonged hypotony because of accompanying ciliary detachment.

Inflammation produces an accumulation of fluid in the suprachoroidal space. The protein concentration in choroidal detachment is about 60% of that of plasma but is otherwise similar in colloidal constituents to plasma, which suggests that the suprachoroidal fluid originates in the choroidal vessels [7]. Further, inflammation increases extravasation, leading to choroidal detachment.

13.4.2 Management of Choroidal Detachment

Management of choroidal detachment consists of medical therapy and surgical therapy.

13.4.2.1 Conservative/Medical Therapy

When the choroidal detachment is small and the anterior chamber is deep or slightly shallow, it is usually best to carefully observe before intervening, since the majority of choroidal detachments resolve within 1–2 weeks, or whenever the IOP reaches 5–7 mmHg.

Compression bandaging to increase IOP may be indicated where there is excessive filtration. Alternatively, intracameral injection of viscoelastic material can be used to maintain the anterior chamber and increase IOP. However, excessive use of viscoelastic material can lead to abnormal IOP elevation and, where choroidal detachment

is the main cause of shallow anterior chamber, it can be difficult to inject the viscoelastic material to sufficiently deepen the anterior chamber.

Because intraocular inflammation may play a role in the development of choroidal detachment, the use of corticosteroids, used either topically or systemically, should be considered, especially in cases of moderate to severe postoperative inflammation.

Hyperosmotic agents and also be useful, by reducing the size of the choroidal detachment and deepening the anterior chamber. Thus, in cases of large choroidal detachment, such agents are drip-infused intravenously.

13.4.2.2 Surgical Therapy

In cases where loose sutures of the scleral flap may have contributed to the hypotony, additional sutures to the scleral flap are recommended. It is also recommended to use additional sutures in the conjunctiva where bleb leakage is present.

Although it is rare, kissing choroidal detachment is a serious condition requiring prompt intervention. In this condition, the anterior chamber is often absent or extremely shallow. When all conservative and medical measures are ineffective, choroidal drainage is the treatment of choice. After dissecting the conjunctiva, sclerostomy is performed by surgical knife approximately 6–9 mm from the limbus. The eyeball is then gently pressed to expel subchoroidal fluid from the eye. This fluid is usually clear, yellow-colored, and non-viscous (Fig. 13.7). While this

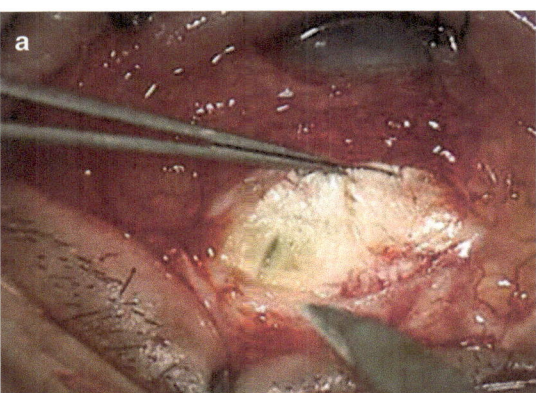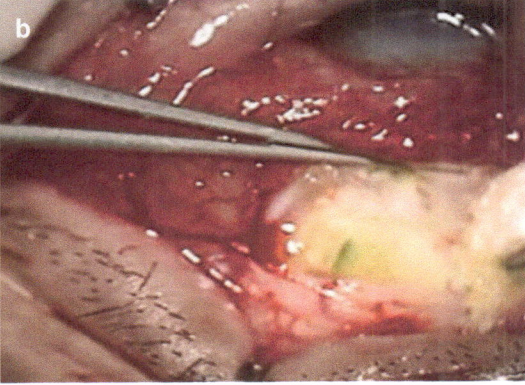

Fig. 13.7 Drainage of choroidal fluid. (**a**) Sclera is dissected using a surgical knife. (**b**) Subchoroidal fluid is expelled from the eye, appearing transparent and yellow-colored

procedure is effective in eliminating choroidal detachment, it is often accompanied by flattening of the filtering bleb following the choroidal drainage.

13.5 Summary

Appropriate management of early postoperative complications, such as malignant glaucoma and choroidal detachment, is key to the success of drainage surgery, including trabeculectomy, especially in eyes with primary angle-closure disease.

Declaration of any potential financial and non-financial conflicts of interest.

Conflicts of Interest: T. Yamamoto, Grant Support (Alcon Japan, Alcon Pharma, Otsuka, Pfizer, Santen, Senju), Consultant/Advisor (Alcon Japan, Alcon Pharma, Astellas Pharma, Kowa, Otsuka, Pfizer, pH Pharma, Rohto, Santen, Seed, Senju), Lecture Fees (Alcon Japan, Alcon Pharma, Johnson & Johnson, Kowa, Novartis, Otsuka, Pfizer, Santen, Senju).

References

1. Chandler PA. Malignant glaucoma. Am J Ophthalmol. 1951;34:993–1000.
2. He F, Qian Z, Lu L, Jiang J, Fan X, Wang Z, Xu X. Clinical efficacy of modified partial pars plana vitrectomy combined with phacoemulsification for malignant glaucoma. Eye (Lond). 2016;30:1094–100. https://doi.org/10.1038/eye.2016.106.
3. Balekudaru S, Choudhari NS, Rewri P, George R, Bhende PS, Bhende M, et al. Surgical management of malignant glaucoma: a retrospective analysis of fifty eight eyes. Eye (Lond). 2017;31:947–55. https://doi.org/10.1038/eye.2017.32.
4. Dave P, Senthil S, Rao HL, Garudadri CS. Treatment outcomes in malignant glaucoma. Ophthalmology. 2013;120:984–90. https://doi.org/10.1016/j.ophtha.2012.10.024.
5. Yamashita H, Eguchi S, Yamamoto T, Shirato S, Kitazawa Y. Trabeculectomy: a prospective study of complications and results of long-term follow-up. Jpn J Ophthalmol. 1985;29:250–62.
6. Brubaker RF, Pederson JE. Choroidal detachment. Surv Ophthalmol. 1983;27:281–9.
7. Chylack LT Jr, Bellows AR. Molecular sieving in in suprachoroidal fluid formation in man. Invest Ophthalmol Vis Sci. 1978;17:420–7.

Management of Acute Primary Angle Closure

Yan Shi and Ningli Wang

Abstract

Acute primary angle-closure (APAC) develops due to abrupt occlusion of the drainage angle by iris tissues. It has serious long-term consequences and is potentially blinding. Our understanding of the pathogenesis of primary angle-closure glaucoma (PACG) has been improved in recent years. The ocular anatomic differences exist between acute and chronic PACG cases, which suggest that the management of acute and chronic PACG differs considerably. A logical approach in the management of APAC can be summarized as an initial lowering of intraocular pressure (IOP), relieving pupil block, and advanced measures for a permanent solution. Timely control of IOP is crucial not only for preventing visual loss from the high-pressure episode but also for preventing progression to chronic angle-closure glaucoma (CACG). For many years, treatment has included medical therapy and laser peripheral iridotomy (LPI) as primary treatment. As lens extraction has become a safer, faster, and more affordable procedure, its role in the treatment of angle closure is coming to the forefront. Combined with goniosynechiolysis, phacoemulsification surgery was considered as a useful and practical method to treat refractory APAC. However, emergency phacoemulsification surgery on inflamed "hot" eyes with high IOP is challenging, and so does trabeculectomy, which has a limited role in an acute setting with numerous possible complications. Controlled diode laser transscleral cyclophotocoagulation plus intracameral triamcinolone acetonide is probably a quick and safe alternative strategy to quiet the inflamed eye, then give a longer time-limited window for sequential surgeries for a permanent solution. Nevertheless, ophthalmologists need to interpret all the results of the present interventions with critical thinking and formulate individualized treatment plans for each patient.

Keywords

Acute primary angle closure
Laser peripheral iridotomy · Cataract surgery
Goniosynechiolysis · Trabeculectomy
Diode laser transscleral cyclophotocoagulation

Y. Shi
Beijing Tongren Eye Center, Beijing Tongren Hospital, Capital Medical University, Beijing, China

N. Wang (✉)
Beijing Tongren Eye Center, Beijing Tongren Hospital, Beijing Institute of Ophthalmology, Capital Medical University, Beijing, China
e-mail: wningli@vip.163.com

Acute primary angle closure (APAC) is a severe and symptomatic ocular hypertension caused by the abrupt closure of the anterior chamber angle. It is also called an acute angle-closure crisis (AACC), because it was an ophthalmic emergency, with an urgent necessity to lower intraocular pressures (IOP) to prevent visual loss. It is common in East Asian people, with a reported prevalence of 1.5% in Guangzhou Chinese 50 years or older, [1, 2] and incidence of 10.4 per 100,000 per year in 30 years or older population in Hong Kong, [3] and 12.2 per 100,000 per year in Singapore [4]. Of these, it estimated that visual acuity (VA) worse than 20/40 was noted in 58% of eyes while 11.4–18%were blinded [5, 6]. Therefore, the appropriate clinical management of APAC is of critical importance to reducing glaucoma blindness.

14.1 Pathogenesis

The pathogenesis of angle closure has been evolving as the imaging devices for the anterior segment of the eye developed in recent years. Aside from pupillary block and plateau iris, multiple mechanisms are recognized as more common contributors for the closure of the angle. More and more studies confirmed that the configuration and dynamic behavior of the iris, ciliary body, and choroid may be responsible for the presenting features of primary angle-closure glaucoma (PACG) [7–12]. The dynamic behavior of the uvea (including iris, ciliary body, and choroid) may also have something to do with sympathetic-parasympathetic nerve activity, especially in APAC, because IOP can be affected by the emotional state [13, 14].

Recent Genome-Wide Association Studies also identified several new PACG loci and genes, which may shed light on the molecular mechanisms of PACG and support the pathogenesis of uvea on PACG. Study has revealed the contributing role of ABCC5 (ATP binding cassette subfamily C member 5) in the normal variation of anterior chamber depth (ACD), a quantitative trait of anatomical risk factor for PACG [15]. Another study showed that EPDR1

(ependymin related 1) was associated with the cell adhesion and choroidal expansion, a highly possible critical pathogenic factor in PACG although its exact role has still not been identified [16]. CHAT has a role in pupillary and ciliary muscle constriction [16].

Notably, the crucial role of the lens in the pathogenesis of angle-closure disease was largely revealed. It was believed that either an increase in its thickness or a more anterior position resulted in angle crowding and a greater predisposition to pupillary block [9, 17].

According to all the new findings in pathogenesis, the classification of PACG can further be divided into five types (Fig. 14.1): pupillary block, [18] plateau iris, [19] anteriorly rotated ciliary body, [20, 21] changes in lens position [20] and choroidal expansion [22]. It was reported that 54.8% PACG in Chinese patients was caused by multiple mechanisms, 38.1% was caused by pure pupillary block and less than 7.1% was caused by pure non-pupillary block mechanisms [23]. Therefore, non-pupillary block factors should still be evaluated and handled after the relief of the pupillary block.

Moreover, APAC had different ocular anatomies compared with chronic primary angle-closure glaucoma (PACG) cases, such as a less deep anterior chamber, thicker lens, shorter axis, and more narrow entrance of chamber angle. Meanwhile, acute cases are more common for females, while chronic cases are more common for males [24]. These differences also suggested that the management of acute and chronic PACG differs considerably.

14.2 Management of APAC

In clinical practice, APAC can be further divided into preclinical, attack (including acute, subacute, or intermediate attacks), intermittent, chronic progression, and absolute stages according to the symptom and signs [25, 26]. Therefore, timely control of IOP is crucial not only for preventing visual loss but also for preventing progression to chronic angle-closure glaucoma (CACG). As an important cause of blindness in

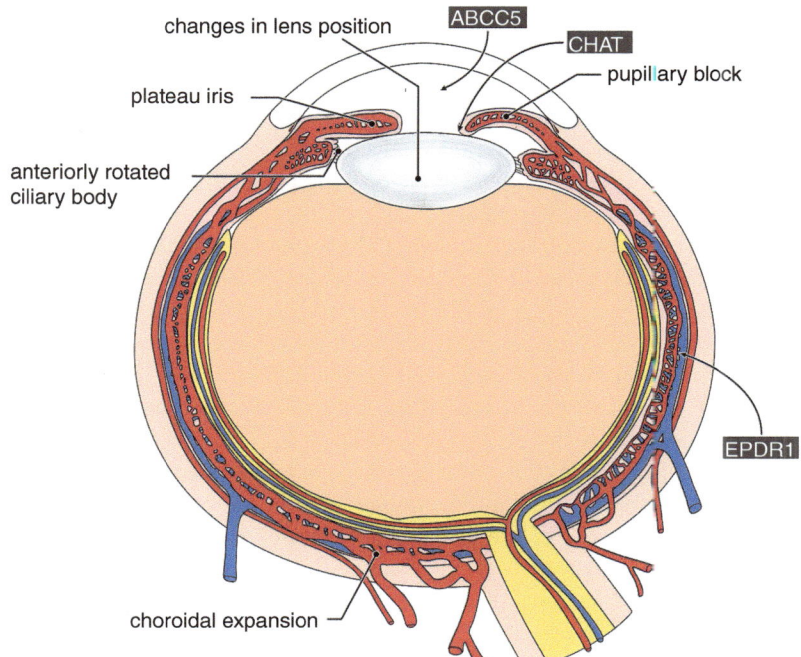

Fig. 14.1 the illustration of the pathogenesis of new primary angle-closure glaucoma (PACG) genes and associated classification of PACG

East Asian people, it was reported that 18% of eyes had become blind, 48% of eyes had developed glaucomatous optic neuropathy, and 58% of eyes had vision worse than 20/40 in the 4–10 years following an acute attack [6].

Traditional initial treatment for APAC includes the use of IOP–lowering medications followed by relief of pupillary block by laser peripheral iridotomy (LPI)/argon laser peripheral iridoplasty (ALPI) [27, 28]. Despite initial successes, it was reported that 38–58.1% of patients had persistently raised IOP subsequently need ocular hypotensive medications in the long term, with 32.7% eventually requiring trabeculectomy [6, 27, 29]. The reasons include an extensive residual appositional closure after LPI, potentially as a result of an anteriorly positioned ciliary body, [30] or direct trabeculum damage and extensive peripheral anterior synechiae (PAS) as a result of the inflammatory response or prolonged angle closure during the acute attack [30]. Therefore, the treatment aims to lower IOP as quickly as possible in order to allow resolution of the corneal edema and alleviate the inflammation on the "hot eye," followed by some form of surgical intervention for a permanent solution, thereby

lowering the possibility of causing irreversible damage to the optic nerve head and other anterior segment structures, and avoiding recurrent attacks and retard progression to CACG [31]. Hence, the protocol for the management of APAC can be summarized as an initial lowering of IOP, relieving pupil block, and advanced measures for a permanent solution.

14.3   Initial Lowering of IOP

The conventional practice in the initial lowering of the pressure involves topical and systemic medical therapy. For those refractory to medical therapy, anterior chamber paracentesis will be introduced. There are still some alternative strategies, such as anterior chamber paracentesis, ALPI and argon laser pupilloplasty, corneal indentation.

14.3.1 Medical Therapy

Systemic medication and various combinations of IOP-lowering agents are usually adopted in conventional treatment, with topical steroids used for the control of intraocular inflammation, which could probably reduce the iris synechia. Concerns of usage of pilocarpine were addressed before. It is intended to be used to induce pupillary constriction, and then lead to the opening of the narrow angle and thus facilitates aqueous outflow. However, its effects of causing shallowing of the anterior chamber by increasing axial lens thickness and inducing anterior lens movement might worsen the situation, especially in eyes with fixed dilated pupil, which presents iris sphincter ischemia and paralysis at high IOP [32–34]. It is known as the paradoxical reaction to pilocarpine [35, 36]. And it was recommended to be given 1 h after the initial reduction of IOP to wait for the recovery of the iris sphincter from ischemia and paralysis.

With medical therapy, it was reported that APAC attacks resolved within 3, 6, 12, and 24 h in 21.5%, 44.6%, 76.2%, and 89.2% subjects, respectively [37]. Therefore, it remains the mainstay of first-line therapy for APAC due to its relative safety and efficacy.

14.3.2 Anterior Chamber Paracentesis

IOP lowers more rapidly with anterior chamber (AC) paracentesis in comparison with conventional medical treatment. However, the IOP-lowering effect of AC paracentesis is short-lived, and repeat treatments are frequently required unless further treatment is intervened [38, 39]. Therefore, it may be best considered as a temporizing measure until definitive treatment is instituted [40]. Meanwhile, considering patients' discomfort to cooperate, or the complications such as damage to the surrounding corneal endothelium, iris, or lens, malignant glaucoma, suprachoroidal hemorrhage, decompression retinopathy, hyphema, and endophthalmitis, it is important to take caution when using AC paracentesis [39]. Currently, as an easy approach in the ophthalmic emergency basis, it remains as surgery for patients for whom medical therapy is either unavailable or unresolvable. After AC

paracentesis, LPI usually could be done in eyes with the clear cornea. Otherwise, the next option would be to perform a surgical iridectomy [41].

14.3.3 Other Strategies

Some studies have shown the efficacy of other IOP-lowering strategies for APAC, such as ALPI [42, 43], argon laser pupilloplasty [44], and corneal indentation [45–47]. However, taking into account the various difficulties associated with their usages, these may not be widely accepted in practice. For ALPI or argon laser pupilloplasty, one possible limitation is that APAC patients are often presented at the emergency room at night, doctors with sufficient skill to perform these procedures may be not available. For corneal indentation, people may concern that the effect of raised IOP during the process of indentation could aggravate ischemic damage to ocular tissues [47]. Lying the patient supine might also work occasionally as in such position, the lens-iris diaphragm would be able to move posteriorly with gravity, which may particularly useful in such instances where there is zonular instability. Occasionally, even corneal scraping was attempted to scrape off with a needle under topical anesthesia to create an area of the clear cornea through which an LPI may be attempted. While these strategies can just be used as a temporizing measure and also be used in conjunction with any of the other procedures, so as to achieve a quicker clearance of corneal edema prior to LPI [41].

14.4 Relieving Pupil Block

14.4.1 LPI

After the initial treatment, the acute attack could be aborted in most cases. However, the rate of recurrence of another acute attack is high unless definitive treatment is performed. Once the IOP has been lower sufficiently to allow corneal edema to clear, LPI will be introduced. LPI has been established as a safe and effective treatment for APAC to relieve pupil block and has supersed surgical peripheral iridectomy due to its non-invasive nature, ease of performing the procedure on an outpatient basis, and the low risk of complications [27]. Although Caucasian eyes usually benefit from LPI alone, the ethnic difference in IOP outcome does exist in Asian eyes. A subsequent rise in IOP is seen in 76.6% of Asian eyes within the first 6 months of the acute attack, and 58.2% still require the use of additional anti-glaucoma medication/filtration surgery to control IOP [48]. Moreover, prophylactic treatment with LPI is required and particularly effective in almost completely preventing an APAC attack in the fellow eye, half of which will otherwise suffer an acute attack within 5 years [27].

14.4.2 Lens Extraction or Phacoemulsification With/Without Goniosynechiolysis

Traditionally, filtration surgery (trabeculectomy) is a viable option for cases refractory to above standard therapies, possibly with combined lens extraction if warranted [49]. While lens extraction alone has been shown to be effective in the treatment of unresponsive APAC patients [50, 51]. Removal of the thick lens in APAC could increase the depth of the anterior chamber, relieve the pupil block and even resolve the anterior-placed ciliary processes, and then markedly decreases angle crowding, thus widening the angle [52–54]. Its popularity in APAC management has followed the technological advances in small-incision cataract surgery and the increasing expertise amongst the surgeons, especially the technique of phacoemulsification, therefore, it has gradually become a much more viable option.

There has been a study revealing that phacoemulsification of lens with intraocular lens (IOL) implantation procedure itself and the use of viscoelastic deepen the anterior chamber intraoperatively would both lead to the breakdown of PAS to a certain extent (PAS > 270-degree, reduced from 43% preoperatively to 24% postoperatively) [55]. Hence, treatment directed at breaking PAS in combination with cataract surgery, such as phacoemulsification combined with gonio-

synechiolysis, was thought to be a feasible option for the treatment of refractory APAC prior to considering filtration surgery.

The goniosynechiolysis can be performed either by knife or by injecting viscoelastic after phacoemulsification. By using the blunt Swan knife, the angle structures were posteriorly pressed until the trabecular meshwork being revisualized under direct visualization with a goniolens. It was reported that this technique could reduce PAS from 310° to 60° with no recurrence of PAS up to 6 years in patients with APAC unresponsive to LPI/ALPI, and the success rate for IOP control was up to 90.4% (mean IOP ≤ 20 mmHg without need for additional medication) [56]. Complications of this procedure include fibrinoid anterior chamber reaction, photophobia, transient elevation of IOP, hyphema, and iridodialysis [56, 57]. While viscogoniosynechiolysis is also effective in the removal of PAS, which is performed by injecting viscoelastic near the angle after IOL implantation with/without direct visualization with a goniolens. Compared with the surgical viscogoniosynechiolysis, it is less traumatic and hence results in fewer complications [58]. However, critics may argue that goniosynechiolysis with simple viscoelastic is not strong enough to resolve the more established, adhesive segments of PAS [41].

14.5 Advanced Measures

14.5.1 Trabeculectomy/Phacotrabeculectomy

Filtration surgery in the form of trabeculectomy alone or combined cataract extraction is usually reserved as the final step in the management of APAC when the condition has been refractory to all other modalities of treatment. Regarding the hot and inflamed nature of the APAC eye with the unbroken acute attack, the complications of primary trabeculectomy in these eyes are numerous and can be sight threatening with serious consequences, including shallow or flat anterior chamber, malignant glaucoma, suprachoroidal hemorrhage, hypotony with resultant maculopathy, bleb leak, blebitis, and endophthalmitis [59–61]. The risk of complications, including endophthalmitis, over filtration, and hypotony, might increase as a result of adopting adjunctive antifibrotic agents such as mitomycin C [62–65].

Moreover, its efficacy was also a concern, as its success (defined as reducing IOP to 22 mmHg) rate in a study of trabeculectomy in patients with medically unresponsive APAC was revealed to be only 56.2%, while the success rate reached 70–95% when trabeculectomy was used conventionally for treatment of a quiet eye with CACG [66]. The indication for performing trabeculectomy surgery may only include those that had an acute on chronic type of presentation, where there was already extensive damage to the optic nerve and/or the persistence of high IOP after other treatments such as LPI [41].

14.5.2 Diode Laser Transscleral Cyclophotocoagulation (DLTSCP)

Phacoemulsification and trabeculectomy/phacotrabeculectomy may a permanent solution to most APAC. However, emergency phacoemulsification or trabeculectomy surgery in APAC on inflamed "hot" eyes with high IOP is challenging, [53, 66] with a poor intraoperative view conferring increased risk of operative complications (such as corneal endothelial damage/posterior capsular rupture, etc.) and sudden ocular decompression from a high starting IOP risking suprachoroidal hemorrhage and permanent visual loss [66–68]. Moreover, uncontrolled IOP at the time of trabeculectomy surgery in patients with APAC is associated with an increased risk of failure (approximately 35%) [66]. For inflamed eyes, topical anesthesia may not be an optimal option, and the risk of postoperative complications would be higher. Therefore, the timing of these interventions in an acute setting would be crucial, and it is essential to take into consideration the need for acute IOP lowering as soon as possible against surgery in an inflamed edematous eye [53].

DLTSCP, initially reserved for eyes with refractory glaucoma and limited visual progno-sis, is now being used more widely, even as primary surgical treatment in glaucoma therapy, including primary open-angle and pseudoexfoliative glaucoma, [69, 70] chronic angle-closure glaucoma, [71, 72] and even eyes with good vision [73]. Recently, DLTSCP followed by lensectomy/combined phacotrabeculectomy has been also described as a safe and effective management strategy in APAC refractory to medical therapies to achieve IOP control [74, 75]. No intraoperative complications were reported during delayed lensectomy after IOP control had been instituted [74]. The only adverse event reported is mild anterior uveitis that occurred 14 months after presentation. It is possible that the inflammation was related to the higher laser energy used [75].

In authors' clinical practice, controlled TSCP with only 5–10 pop effects on the ciliary body combined with intracameral triamcinolone acetonide (1 mg) succeeded to create exudative detachment of the ciliary body on these "hot" eyes, after that, the IOP decreased to around 10 mmHg and lasted for 7–14 days, and the anterior chamber deepened with minimal inflammation. Then the sequential phacoemulsification with viscogoniosynechiolysis could be performed with no complications on these "quiet eye."

14.6 Conclusions

The appropriate clinical management of APAC is of critical importance to reducing glaucoma blindness. Acute IOP lowering was crucial for avoiding visual loss from the high-pressure episode and preventing progression to chronic angle-closure glaucoma (CACG). For many years, treatment has included medical therapy and LPI as primary treatment. However, as lens extraction has become a safer, faster, and more affordable procedure, its role in the treatment of angle closure is coming to the forefront. Moreover, the timing of any sequential surgeries should also consider the technical difficulties during surgery and postoperative complications in these inflamed edematous eyes.

Ophthalmologists need to interpret all the results of the present interventions with critical thinking and formulate individualized treatment plans for each patient.

References

1. He M, Foster PJ, Ge J, Huang W, Zheng Y, Friedman DS, et al. Prevalence and clinical characteristics of glaucoma in adult Chinese: a population-based study in Liwan District. Guangzhou Invest Ophthalmol Vis Sci. 2006;47(7):2782–8.
2. Foster PJ, Oen FT, Machin D, Ng TP, Devereux JG, Johnson GJ, et al. The prevalence of glaucoma in Chinese residents of Singapore: a cross-sectional population survey of the Tanjong Pagar district. Arch Ophthalmol. 2000;118(8):1105–11.
3. Lai JS, Liu DT, Tham CC, Li RT, Lam DS. Epidemiology of acute primary angle-closure glaucoma in the Hong Kong Chinese population: prospective study. Hong Kong Med J. 2001;7(2):118–23.
4. Seah SKL, Foster PJ, Chew PTK, Jap A, Oen F, Han BF, et al. Incidence of acute primary angle-closure Glaucoma in Singapore: an island-wide survey. Arch Ophthalmol. 1997;115(11):1436–40.
5. Lee JW, Wong BK, Yick DW, Wong IY, Yuen CY, Lai JS. Primary acute angle closure: long-term clinical outcomes over a 10-year period in the Chinese population. Int Ophthalmol. 2014;34(2):165–9.
6. Aung T, Friedman DS, Chew PT, Ang LP, Gazzard G, Lai YF, et al. Long-term outcomes in Asians after acute primary angle closure. Ophthalmology. 2004;111(8):1464–9.
7. Ye Z, Zhen LS, Lei L, Guang HM, Ravi T, Li WN. Quantitative analysis of iris changes after physiologic and pharmacologic mydriasis in a rural Chinese population. Invest Ophthalmol Vis Sci. 2014;55(7):4405–12.
8. Li S, Jiang J, Yang Y, Wu G, Li SM, Thomas R, et al. Pupil size associated with the largest Iris volume in Normal Chinese eyes. J Ophthalmol. 2018;2018:8058951.
9. Marchini G, Pagliarusco A, Toscano A, Tosi R, Brunelli C, Bonomi L. Ultrasound biomicroscopic and conventional ultrasonographic study of ocular dimensions in primary angle-closure glaucoma. Ophthalmology. 1998;105(11):2091–8.
10. Zhang Y, Li SZ, Li L, He MG, Thomas R, Wang NL. Dynamic Iris changes as a risk factor in primary angle closure disease. Invest Ophthalmol Vis Sci. 2016;57(1):218–26.
11. Wang YX, Ran J, Xiao LR, Jian DC, Hong LS, Liang X, et al. Intraocular pressure elevation and choroidal thinning. Br J Ophthalmol. 2016;100(12):1676–81.
12. Gao K, Li F, Li Y, Li X, Huang W, Chen S, et al. Anterior Choroidal thickness increased in primary open-angle Glaucoma and primary angle-closure

disease eyes evidenced by ultrasound biomicroscopy and SS-OCT. Invest Ophthalmol Vis Sci. 2018;59(3):1270–7.
13. Shily BG. Psychophysiological stress, elevated intraocular pressure, and acute closed-angle glaucoma. Am J Optom Physiol Optic. 1987;64(11):866–70.
14. Kong X, Yan M, Sun X, Xiao Z. Anxiety and depression are more prevalent in primary angle closure glaucoma than in primary open-angle glaucoma. J Glaucoma. 2013;24(5):e57–63.
15. Nongpiur ME, Khor CC, Jia H, Corres BK, Chen LJ, Qiao C, et al. ABCC5, a gene that influences the anterior chamber depth, is associated with primary angle closure glaucoma. PLoS Genet. 2014;10(3):e1004089.
16. Khor CC, Do T, Jia H, Nakano M, George R, Abu-Amero K, et al. Genome-wide association study identifies five new susceptibility loci for primary angle closure glaucoma. Nat Genet. 2016;48(5):556–62.
17. Nongpiur ME, Mingguang H, Nishani A, Friedman DS, Wan-Ting T, Mani B, et al. Lens vault, thickness, and position in Chinese subjects with angle closure. Ophthalmology. 2011;118(3):474–9.
18. Tarongoy P, Ho CL, Walton DS. Angle-closure Glaucoma: the role of the lens in the pathogenesis, prevention, and treatment. Surv Ophthalmol. 2009;54(2):211–25.
19. Wang N, Ouyang J, Zhou W. Multiple patterns of angle closure mechanisms in primary angle closure glaucoma in Chinese. Zhonghua Yan Ke Za Zhi 2000 Jan;36(1):46-51, 5, 6.
20. Ng WT, Morgan W. Mechanisms and treatment of primary angle closure: a review. Clin Exp Ophthalmol. 2012;40(4):e218–28.
21. Liebmann JM, Weinreb RN, Ritch R. Angle-closure glaucoma associated with occult annular ciliary body detachment. Arch Ophthalmol. 1998.116(6):731–5.
22. Nickla DL, Wallman J. The multifunctional choroid. Prog Retin Eye Res. 2010;29(2):144–68.
23. Wang N, Heping WU, Fan Z, Center ZO, University Z, Guangzhou. Primary angle closure glaucoma in Chinese and Western populations. Chin Med J. 2002;115(11):1706–15.
24. Sun X, Ji X, Zheng Y. Primary chronic angle-closure Glaucoma in Chinese—a clinical exploration of its pathogenesis and natural course. Yan Ke Xue Bao. 1994;10(3):176–85.
25. Ji X, Yuan S, Chen S, Guo B. Clinical natural course of congestive glaucoma. Chin J Ophthalmol. 1966;13:78–80.
26. Salmon JF. The role of trabeculectomy in the treatment of advanced chronic angle-closure glaucoma. J Glaucoma. 1993;2(4):285–90.
27. Aung T, Ang LP, Chan SP, Chew PT. Acute primary angle-closure: long-term intraocular pressure outcome in Asian eyes. Am J Ophthalmol. 2001;131(1):7–12.
28. Robin AL, Pollack IP. Argon laser peripheral iridotomies in the treatment of primary angle closure glaucoma. Long-term follow-up. Arch Ophthalmol. 1982;100(6):919–23.

29. Lam DS, Lai JS, Tham CC, Chua JK, et al. Argon laser peripheral iridoplasty versus conventional systemic medical therapy in treatment of acute primary angle-closure glaucoma: a prospective, randomized, controlled trial. Ophthalmology. 2002;109(9):1591–6.
30. Yeung BYM, Ng PWC, Chiu TYH, Wai TC, Li FCH, Chung Chai C, et al. Prevalence and mechanism of appositional angle closure in acute primary angle closure after iridotomy. Australian & New Zealand J Ophthalmol. 2010;33(5):478–82.
31. David R, ., Tessler Z, ., Yassur Y, . Long-term outcome of primary acute angle-closure glaucoma. Br J Ophthalmol 1985;69(4):261–262.
32. Abramson DH, Chang S, ., Coleman DJ, Smith ME. Pilocarpine-induced lens changes. An ultrasonic biometric evaluation of dose response. Arch Ophthalmol 1974;92(6):464–469.
33. Abramson DH, Coleman DJ, Forbes M, ., Franzen LA. Pilocarpine. Effect on the anterior chamber and lens thickness. Arch Ophthalmol 1972;87(6):615–620.
34. Wilkie J, Drance SM, Schulzer M. The effects of Miotics on anterior-chamber depth. Am J Ophthalmol. 1969;68(1):78–83.
35. Bleiman BS, Schwartz AL. Paradoxical intraocular pressure response to pilocarpine. A proposed mechanism and treatment. Arch Ophthalmol. 1979;97(7):1305–6.
36. Ritch R. The Pilocarpine paradox. J Glaucoma. 1996;5(4):225–7.
37. Ramli N, Chai SM, Tan GS, Husain R, S-T H, C-L H, et al. Efficacy of medical therapy in the initial management of acute primary angle closure in Asians. Eye. 2010;24(10):1599–602.
38. Lam DSC, Tham CCY, Lai JSM, DYL L. Current approaches to the management of acute primary angle closure. Cur Opin Ophthalmol. 2007;18(2):146–51.
39. Lam DSC, Chua JKH, Tham CCY, Lai JSM. Efficacy and safety of immediate anterior chamber paracentesis in the treatment of acute primary angle-closure glaucoma: a pilot study 1. Ophthalmology. 2002;109(1):64–70.
40. Pong JCF. Anterior chamber paracentesis in patients with acute elevation of intraocular pressure. Graefes Arch Clin Exp Ophthalmol. 2008;246(3):463–4. author reply 5-6
41. Boey PY, Singhal S, Perera SA, Aung T. Conventional and emerging treatments in the management of acute primary angle closure. Clin Ophthalmol. 2012;6:417–24.
42. Lam DSC, Lai JSM, Tham CCY, Chua JKH, Poon ASY. Argon laser peripheral iridoplasty versus conventional systemic medical therapy in treatment of acute primary angle-closure glaucoma: a prospective, randomized, controlled trial. Ophthalmology. 2002;109(9):1591–6.
43. Lam DS, Lai JS, Tham CC. Immediate argon laser peripheral iridoplasty as treatment for acute attack of primary angle-closure glaucoma: a preliminary study. Ophthalmology. 1998;105(12):2231–6.

44. Robert Ritch MD. Argon laser treatment for medically unresponsive attacks of angle-closure Glaucoma. Am J Ophthalmol. 1982;94(2):197–204.
45. Anderson DR. Corneal indentation to relieve acute angle-closure glaucoma. Am J Ophthalmol. 1979;88(6):1091–3.
46. Masselos K, Bank A, Francis IC, Stapleton F. Corneal indentation in the early management of acute angle closure. Ophthalmology. 2009;116(1):25–9.
47. Teichmann KD. Corneal indentation to relieve glaucoma. Am J Ophthalmol. 1980;90(3):434–5.
48. Fleck BW, Wright E, Fairley EA. A randomised prospective comparison of operative peripheral iridectomy and Nd:YAG laser iridotomy treatment of acute angle closure glaucoma: 3 year visual acuity and intraocular pressure control outcome. Br J Ophthalmol. 1997;81(10):884–8.
49. Lai JSM, Tham CCY, Lam DSC. Incisional surgery for angle closure glaucoma. Semin Ophthalmol. 2002;17(2):92–9.
50. Jacobi PC, Dietlein TS, Lüke C, Engels B, Krieglstein GK. Primary phacoemulsification and intraocular lens implantation for acute angle-closure glaucoma. Ophthalmology. 2002;109(9):1597–603.
51. Lam DS, Leung DY, Tham CC, Li FC, Kwong YY, Chiu TY, et al. Randomized trial of early phacoemulsification versus peripheral iridotomy to prevent intraocular pressure rise after acute primary angle closure. Ophthalmology. 2008;115(7):1134–40.
52. Tarongoy P, Ho CL, Walton DS. Angle-closure glaucoma: the role of the lens in the pathogenesis, prevention, and treatment. Surv Ophthalmol. 2009;54(2):211–25.
53. Tan GS, Hoh ST, Husain R, Gazzard G, Oen FT, Seah SK, et al. Visual acuity after acute primary angle closure and considerations for primary lens extraction. Br J Ophthalmol. 2006;90(1):14–6.
54. Atsushi N, Takehisa K, Masashi K, Kenji Y, Masashi F, Takuji I, et al. Angle widening and alteration of ciliary process configuration after cataract surgery for primary angle closure. Ophthalmology. 2006;113(3):437–41.
55. Lai JS, Tham CC, Chan JC. The clinical outcomes of cataract extraction by phacoemulsification in eyes with primary angle-closure glaucoma (PACG) and co-existing cataract: a prospective case series. J Glaucoma. 2006;15(1):47–52.
56. Teekhasaenee C, Ritch R. Combined phacoemulsification and goniosynechialysis for uncontrolled chronic angle-closure glaucoma after acute angle-closure glaucoma. Ophthalmology. 1999;106(4):669–74.
57. Lai JS, Tham CC, Lam DS. The efficacy and safety of combined phacoemulsification, intraocular lens implantation, and limited goniosynechialysis, followed by diode laser peripheral iridoplasty, in the treatment of cataract and chronic angle-closure glaucoma. J Glaucoma. 2001;10(4):309–15.
58. Varma D, Baylis O, Wride N, Phelan PS, Fraser SG. Viscogonioplasty: an effective procedure for low-

ering intraocular pressure in primary angle closure glaucoma. Eye. 2007;21(4):472–5.

59. Bellucci R, Perfetti S, Babighian S, Morselli S, Bonomi L. Filtration and complications after trabeculectomy and after phaco-trabeculectomy. Acta Ophthalmol Scand Suppl. 2010;75(S224):44–5.

60. Membrey WL, Poinoosawmy DP, Bunce C, Hitchings RA. Glaucoma surgery with or without adjunctive antiproliferatives in normal tension glaucoma: 1 intraocular pressure control and complications. Br J Ophthalmol. 2000;84(6):586–90.

61. Costa VP, Smith M, ., Spaeth GL, Gandham S, ., Markovitz B, . Loss of visual acuity after trabeculectomy. Ophthalmology 1993;100(5):599–612.

62. Budenz DL, Pyfer M, Singh K, Gordon J, Piltzseymour J, Keates EU. Comparison of phacotrabeculectomy with 5-fluorouracil, mitomycin-C, and without antifibrotic agents. Ophthalmic Surg Lasers. 1999;30(5):367–74.

63. Yoon PS, Singh K. Update on antifibrotic use in glaucoma surgery, including use in trabeculectomy and glaucoma drainage implants and combined cataract and glaucoma surgery. Curr Opin Ophthalmol. 2004;15(2):141–6.

64. Bindlish R, Condon GP, Schlosser JD, D'Antonio J, Lauer KB, Lehrer R. Efficacy and safety of mitomycin-C in primary trabeculectomy: five-year follow-up. Ophthalmology. 2002;109(7):1336–41.

65. Poulsen EJ, Allingham RR. Characteristics and risk factors of infections after glaucoma filtering surgery. J Glaucoma. 2000;9(6):438–43.

66. Aung T, Tow SL, Yap EY, Chan SP, Seah SK. Trabeculectomy for acute primary angle closure. Ophthalmology. 2001;108(6):1008.

67. Speaker MG, Guerriero PN, Met JA, Coad CT, Berger A, Marmor M. A case-control study of risk factors for intraoperative Suprachoroidal Expulsive hemorrhage. Ophthalmology. 1991;98(2):202–9.

68. Jiraskova N, Rozsival P, Pozlerova J, Ludvikova M, Burova M. Expulsive hemorrhage after glaucoma filtering surgery. Biomed Pap Med Fac Univ Palacky Olomouc Czech Repub. 2009;153(3):221–4.

69. Kramp K, Vick HP, Guthoff R. Transscleral diode laser contact cyclophotocoagulation in the treatment of different glaucomas, also as primary surgery. Graefes Arch Clin Exp Ophthalmol. 2002;240(9):698–703.

70. Grueb M, Rohrbach JM, Bartz-Schmidt KU, Schlote T. Transscleral diode laser cyclophotocoagulation as primary and secondary surgical treatment in primary open-angle and pseudoexfoliatve glaucoma. Long-term clinical outcomes. Graefes Arch Clin Exp Ophthalmol. 2006;244(10):1293–9.

71. Shi Y, Tian J, Han Y, Oatts J, Wang N. Pathogenic role of the vitreous in angle-closure glaucoma with autosomal recessive bestrophinopathy: a case report. BMC Ophthalmol. 2020;20(1):271.

72. Lai JSM, Tham CCY, Chan JCH, Lam DSC. Diode laser transscleral cyclophotocoagulation as primary surgical treatment for medically uncontrolled chronic angle closure glaucoma: long-term clinical outcomes. J Glaucoma. 2005 Apr;14(2):114–9.

73. Ansari E, Gandhewar J. Long-term efficacy and visual acuity following transscleral diode laser photocoagulation in cases of refractory and non-refractory glaucoma. Eye. 2007;21(7):936–40.

74. Manna A, Foster P, Papadopoulos M, Nolan W. Cyclodiode laser in the treatment of acute angle closure. Eye. 2012;26(5):742–5.

75. Yusuf IH, Shah M, Shaikh A, James CB. Transscleral cyclophotocoagulation in refractory acute and chronic angle closure glaucoma. BMJ Case Rep. 2015;2015(3):247–54.

Recent Advances in our
Understanding of the Genetic
Basis of Primary Angle-Closure
Glaucoma

15

Shi Song Rong, Chi Pui Pang, and Li Jia Chen

Abstract

The etiology of primary angle-closure glaucoma (PACG) is multifactorial but much is still to be investigated. Environmental or inducible factors are not evidently identified. Gene variants confirmed in association with PACG account for less than 5% of PACG heritability. Considerably smaller number of genes were mapped and less gene variants known to associate with PACG than primary open-angle glaucoma (POAG), another major form of glaucoma. But PACG loci are clearly distinctive from the associated gene variants of POAG. The genetic components of PACG include large ethnic differences in prevalence, familial trends of occurrence, the heritability of phenotype and susceptible genes which are identified principally by candidate gene investigations, familial linkage analyses, and genome-wide association studies (GWAS). The only PACG endophenotype with known genetic association is anterior chamber depth. More PACG genes will be mapped by GWAS and whole-genome sequencing with family analysis. Genotype-phenotype correlation studies on big cohorts with longitudinal follow up for the establishment of pharmacogenomics database and genetic biomarkers will be key areas of attention for PACG.

Keywords

PACG · Heritability · Ethnicity · Genes Phenotypes

S. S. Rong
Department of Ophthalmology, Harvard Medical School, Massachusetts Eye and Ear, Boston, MA, USA

C. P. Pang
Department of Ophthalmology and Visual Sciences, The Chinese University of Hong Kong, Hong Kong, China
e-mail: cppang@cuhk.edu.hk

L. J. Chen (✉)
Department of Ophthalmology and Visual Sciences, The Chinese University of Hong Kong, Hong Kong, China

Department of Ophthalmology and Visual Sciences, Prince of Wales Hospital, Hong Kong, China
e-mail: lijia_chen@cuhk.edu.hk

15.1 Introduction

Primary angle-closure glaucoma (PACG) is a complex disease with multifactorial etiology, which involves complicated anatomical, physiological and genetic mechanisms [1]. Narrow to closed anterior chamber angle, pupillary block, and plateau iris are essential anatomical features in PACG. The former is a pre-requisite of obstruction to aqueous outflow in the trabecular meshwork. Pupillary block is usually a triggering factor for acute angle-closure attack [2]. The plateau iris is a common cause of persistent occludable angle after iridotomy [3]. PACG is also linked to other anatomical abnormalities, such as shortened axial length, shallowed anterior chamber depth, and increased lens volume as seen in cataract. Environmental risk factors for PACG are not readily quantifiable, except that aging plays an important role. Angle-closure glaucoma (ACG) can be secondary to ocular diseases like chronic uveitis and rubeosis iridis that lead to synechial angle closure. ACG can also develop with some congenital conditions, mainly nanophthalmos and Axenfeld Rieger Syndrome, which are resulted from angle dysgenesis [4–6]. Therefore, there has to be differentiation of primary and secondary forms of ACG for treatment plan since the pathology is so different. The genetic basis for such complex disease mechanisms is understandably complicated [7]. However, in comparison with primary open-angle glaucoma (POAG), another major glaucoma form, there is currently no gene known to cause PACG directly [8]. The number of genes confirmed to have an association with PACG is also limited.

Albeit such complex mechanistic background with unknown environmental risk, the genetic basis of PACG is evidently attributed to ethnic diversities in prevalence, familial linkage, and phenotype heritability [9, 10]. Genes with strong and clear susceptibility for PACG have been mapped by candidate gene approach, family linkage analysis, and genome-wide association study (GWAS) [8, 11].

15.2 Genetic Epidemiology of PACG

PACG prevalence is known to be diversified among different ethnic populations, in general lower in Caucasians and higher in Asian populations [7]. Its occurrence was noticeably high in the Inuit population including Eskimos in the Arctic regions. Almost 5% of the Eskimos populations over 40 years old in Greenland and Alaska have PACG, about 40 times higher than Europeans [12, 13]. In a systemic review of PACG studies in Europeans published during 1948–2011, PACG prevalence for people over 40 years old was 0.4% (95% confidence interval [CI]: 0.3%–0.5%), with female to male ratio 3.25 to 1 [14]. PACG occurs more in Asians than Europeans. In a meta-analysis and review of 50 population-based studies, PACG is the highest in Asia at 1.09% (95% CI: 0.43–2.32%) against 0.60% (95% CI: 0.16–1.48%) in Africa, 0.42% (95% CI: 0.13–0.98%) in Europe, and 0.26% (95% CI: 0.03–0.96%) in North America [15]. When two big Indian studies were included in the meta-analysis, PACG prevalence in Asia was decreased to 0.73% (95% CI: 0.18–1.96%) [16]. It is notable in this study that in contrast to POAG, in which the prevalence is essentially similar among different Asian populations, PACG at age between 40 and 80 years occurs more in East Asia (Mongolia, China, Korea, and Japan) at 1.07% (95% CI: 0.28–2.74%), than South Central Asia (India, Iran, Nepal, and Sri Lanka) at 0.69% (95% CI: 0.13–2.07%) or South East Asia (Singapore, Myanmar, and Thailand) at 0.64% (95% CI: 0.19–1.49%). People in East Asia are 5.55 times (95% CI: 1.52–14.73) more likely than people in South East Asia to develop PACG after adjustment for gender and age [16]. Overall in Asia, males aged between 40 and 80 years have a higher likelihood to have POAG (odds ratio [OR]: 1.37, 95% CI: 1.17–1.59) than females, but less to have PACG (OR: 0.54, 95% CI: 0.41–0.71). For this age range, people of urbanized habitation have less PACG at 0.73% than rural living people at 0.94%. Notably, the trend was reversed for POAG, 2.24% against 1.53%. In a recent study in Eastern India, with 7408 people living in rural areas and 7248 in cities, PACG is also higher in rural living at 1.03% (95% CI: 0.99–1.07%) than in city dwellers at 0.97% (95% CI: 0.94–1.00%) [17].

In Chinese, a meta-analysis of 11 population-based studies conducted in different parts of China during January 1990 to July 2010 involving 35,968 adult Chinese reported a pooled PACG prevalence of 1.4% (95% CI: 1.0–1.7%), with women more likely to have PACG than men (OR: 1.75; 95% CI: 1.20–2.56; $P = 0.004$) [18].

In a recent meta-analysis of 30 cross-sectional studies reported between 1995 and 2016 from various regions of China, PACG prevalence was 1.40% (95% CI: 1.17–1.68%) for Chinese aged between 45 and 89 years [19]. There was also less PACG male patients than females (OR: 0.53; 95% CI: 0.46–0.60) [19]. PACG prevalence was reportedly 0.5% (95% CI: 0.3–0.7%) in a rural population aged over 40 years in the Handan of northern China [20]. In the same population, the prevalence of primary angle closure was higher at 1.5% (95% CI: 1.2–1.8%) and even higher for primary angle-closure suspects at 10.4% (95% CI: 9.6–11.2%). Moreover, females are more likely to develop PACG than males with an OR ranging from 1.75 to 1.89 ($P < 0.05$) [18–20]. Occurrence of POAG was similar, with an overall prevalence at 1.02% (95% CI: 0.67–1.57%) [21].

Ethnic differences in the prevalence of PACG and gender bias in disease susceptibility indicated the presence of genetic influences. In terms of environmental influence, rural living poses a higher risk than urbanized inhabitation.

15.3 Sporadic and Familial PACG

Sporadic PACG is usually late-onset with disease incidence increases with age. Familial history is also long known to be a risk factor across all populations [7, 22, 23]. In Greenland Eskimos, who are Inuit by race, family history poses more than three times risk of PACG [12]. A high heritability of narrow angle of about 60% has been revealed in a study of 100 Chinese probands with 327 first-degree relatives [24]. Among the 515 sibling pairs, a high probability of 50% was detected for narrow angle, with a sevenfold increase in likelihood of narrow angle when compared with the general population.

In 303 South Indian sibling pairs, primary angle closure (PAC)/PACG was found in 11.4% of PAC/PACG siblings but only in 4.9% of primary angle-closure suspects (PACS) siblings ($P = 0.07$) and even none in open-angle (OA) siblings ($P = 0.002$). There was more angle closure in PACS (35.0%) and PAC/PACG siblings (36.7%) than in OA siblings (3.7%; $P < 0.001$).

Multivariable analysis after adjustment for age and gender revealed a 13.6-fold of higher likelihood of having angle closure if one has angle-closure siblings than with OA siblings (95% CI: 4.1–45.0; $P < 0.001$) [25]. In a recent study also in southern India of 636 sibling pairs (482 PACS and 154 PAC/PACG), the occurrence of PAC/PACG among siblings of PAC/PACG was 8.4%, which was higher than the 3.5% of PAC/PACG among siblings of PACS [26]. In Central Asia, familial segregation of angle closure was also reported in an Iranian study, with siblings of PACG patients at higher risk [27].

15.4 Phenotype Heritability

Hereditability of anatomical and ophthalmic features in relation to both major forms of glaucoma, POAG and PACG, have been reported in different ethnic populations. Compared with the general population, PACG has greater central cornea thickness (CCT), shorter axial length (AL), shallower anterior chamber depth (ACD), bigger cup-to-disc ratio, and narrower angle width. These are independent risk factors [17]. Intraocular pressure (IOP) is one dominant risk factor for PACG. Its heritability has been estimated to range from 0.36–0.50 [24, 28]. In Greenland Eskimos, the corneoscleral size was found to be inheritable [13]. For cup-to-disc ratio, the heritability ranged from 0.48 to 0.80 [29, 30]. The variance in drainage angle width in Chinese children appeared to be largely attributable to genetic effects, with a heritability of approximately 70% [31]. The variance of optic nerve head parameters, namely disc area (DA), cup area (CA), and cup/disc area ratio (CDAR) appears to be attributable to additive genetic and unshared environmental effects. Approximately 80% of these phenotypic variances are genetically determined [32]. Genetic variants have been tested in a recent study on Chinese PACG patients, and three SNPs, rs3753841 in *COL11A1*, rs1258267 in *CHAT*, and rs736893 in *GLIS3*, were associated with PACG and also had a mild association with ACD [33]. In the same cohort, rs7290117 in *ZNRF3* was associated with axial length in PACG patients, but not with PACG [34]. Besides, a number of genetic variants associated with the endophenotypes of glaucoma had been identified in population-based samples. A SNP rs1015213 at the *PCMTD1-ST18* locus has been associated with ACD in a European population [35]. SNP rs33912345 in *SIX6*, a POAG gene, has been associated with optic disc parameters in Europeans [36], and retinal nerve fiber layer thickness in Europeans and Chinese [36, 37]. Three SNPs (rs7126851, rs7104512, and rs10835818) in the *ELP4* gene, which neighbors and plays a crucial role in the expression of *PAX6*, were associated with disc area in Caucasians [38]. In a GWAS of optic disc parameters in population-based cohorts, SNPs at chromosomal regions 1p22 (near *CDC7*), 10q21.3-q22.1 (near *ATOH7*), and 16q12.1 were associated with optic disc area, and SNPs at 9p21 (near *CDKN2B*), 14q22.3-q23 (near *SIX1*), 11q13, 13q13, 17q23, and 22q12.1 were associated with vertical cup-to-disc ratio [39].

15.5 Mapping the PACG Genes by Candidate Gene Analysis

Many attempts have been made to map PACG genes in different ethnic populations utilizing cohorts of PACG patients and controls [9]. A candidate gene analysis has led to the identification of nine genes associated with PACG (Table 15.1). In a meta-analysis, we summarized all reported genetic associations from candidate gene analysis and affirmed five genes (*HGF, HSP70, MFRP, MMP9,* and *NOS3*) to be associated with primary angle-closure disease [10]. Most candidate gene association studies did not involve a big sample size. Some of the genes have not been replicated. They are statistically linked to susceptibility to PACG, not directly causative. Understanding of the functions and properties of these genes have given some clues to the disease mechanism but not the elucidation of the pathogenesis [9]. It is notable that *MTHFR* and *HGF* have been linked to the regulation of axial length, and shorter axial length is a trait of PACG.

Different investigation strategies other than direct comparison of patient and control genotypes have recently identified novel PACG genes. In an exploration of gene expressions in peripheral blood of Korean patients with acute PACG, microarray analysis of RNA extracted from mononuclear cells showed upregulation of 347 gene transcripts and downregulation of 696 transcripts by more than twofold than controls. Further molecular studies including RT-PCR have confirmed the association of PACG with thrombospondin-1 (TSP-1), transforming growth factor (TGF-β1), and prostaglandin-endoperoxide synthase (2PGE2) [54]. In a big Iranian pedigree with 8 affected individuals with PAC, confirmed PACG, and PACS, investigations by extensive family linkage analysis, segregation analysis, whole-genome sequencing, and sequence screening of other unrelated patients and controls have identified *COL18A1* mutations evident for causing the iridocorneal angle closure in these patients [53]. Future work on the structural and functional roles of type XVIII collagen, especially in the human iris and cornea, should help to reveal the pathophysiology of angle closure.

15.6 Mapping the PACG Genes by Genome-wide Association Studies

So far three major GWAS have been conducted for PACG, having identified 9 genes with specific polymorphisms associated with PACG with high statistical significance (Table 15.2). The primary cohort was mixed in ethnicities and validation has been conducted in multiple ethnic populations including Caucasians, Indians, Malays, Chinese, Koreans, and Japanese [55, 59, 61]. In a previous meta-analysis, we have assessed replication studies on the GWAS SNPs reported by Vithana E et al. [55] and Nongpiur ME et al. [59], and affirmed 3 of them, rs11024102 of *PLEKHA7*, rs3753841 of *COL11A1* rs1015213 of *PCMTD1-ST18*, to be significantly associated with PACG (Table 15.2) [10]. In subsequent replication studies, three of the associated SNPs, rs1015213 of *PCMTD1-ST18*, rs3816415 of *EPDR1*, and rs3739821 of *DRM2-FAM102A* showed consistent associations with PACS in a

Table 15.1 Candidate genes mapped for primary angle-closure glaucoma

Chromosomal location	Gene	Associated variant	Study population and sample size	Year of report	References
1p36.22	*MTHFR* Methylenetetrahydrofolate reductase	C677T, A1298C	Pakistanis 122 PACG, 143 controls	2009	[40]
		rs1537514 CC genotype	Chinese 232 PACG 306 controls	2016	[41]
2p22.2	*CYP1B1* Cytochrome P450 1B1	(−13 T > C, R48G, A119S, V432L, D449D, and N453S) C-C-G-G-T-A	Indian 90 PACG, 200 controls	2007	[42]
2q32.1	*CALCRL* Calcitonin receptor-like receptor	*CALCRL* gene (AATACAGAT)	Australian Caucasians 107 PACG, 288 controls	2012	[43]
		Haplotype T (rs840617) C (rs6759535) T (rs1157699)	Southern Chinese 207 PACG, 205 controls	2009	[44]
4p16.3	*HGF* Hepatocyte growth factor	rs5745718, rs12536657, rs12540393 and rs17427817	Nepalese 106 PACG, 204 controls	2011	[45]
7q36	eNOS Endothelial nitric oxide synthase	27 bp insertion VNTR intron 4 polymorphism	Pakistanis 111PACG, 166 controls	2010	[46]
		rs3793342 and rs7830 Sex age matched. Bonferroni correction	Australian Caucasians 129 PACG, 288 controls	2013	[47]
		No association	Nepalese 106 PACG, 204 controls	2013	[47]
11q23.3	*MFRP* Membrane type frizzled-related protein	Q175X, 492delC, and I182T, 1143insC	Nanophthalmos Amish-Mennonite kindred, 26 Caucasian kindreds	2005	[4]
		rs3814762	Chinese 232 PACG, 306 controls	2013	[48]
19q13.42	*HSP70* Heat shock protein	rs1043618	Chinese 232 PACG, 306 controls	2013	[48]
		rs1043618 G + 190C	Pakistanis 111PACG, 166 controls	2010	[46]
20q13.12	*MMP9* Matrix metalloproteinase 9	rs3918249, rs17576	Australian Caucasians 107 PACG, 288 controls	2011	[49]
		rs2664538	Taiwan Chinese 78 PACG, 86 controls	2006	[50]
		rs2250889	Southern Chinese 211 PACG, 205 controls	2009	[51]
		rs17576	Pakistanis 82 PACG, 118 controls	2013	[52]
21q22.3	*COL18A1* Collagen XVIIIa1	c.550G > A E184 K	Iranian (Genome-wide SNP genotyping, linkage analysis, segregation analysis, and whole exome sequencing were adopted in this study)	2013	[53]

Table 15.2 PACG susceptible genes identified by Genome-Wide Association Studies

Genes	SNPs	GWAS	GWAS significance	References	Study population	Evaluation significance	References	Meta-analysis significance	References
PLEKHA7	rs11024102	3771 PACG 18,551 controls	OR = 1.23 $P = 3.10 \times 10^{-12}$	[55]	Chinese 1397 PACS 943 controls	Insignificant	[56]	OR = 1.24; $P = 8.3 \times 10^{-5}$	[10]
	rs11024102				Indian 180 PAC/PACG 411 controls	Insignificant	[57]		
COL11A1	rs3753841	3771 PACG 18,551 controls	OR = 1.19 $P = 9.53 \times 10^{-9}$	[55]	Chinese 1397 PACS 943 controls	Insignificant	[56]	OR = 1.22; $P = 4.6 \times 10^{-4}$	[10]
	rs3753841				Australian 232 PACG 288 controls Nepalese 106 PACG 204 controls	$P = 0.009$	[58]		
	rs3753841				Indian 180 PAC/PACG 411 controls	Insignificant	[57]		
	rs1031820				Chinese 232 PACG 306 controls	$P = 0.047$	[41]		
PCMTD1-ST18	rs1015213	3771 PACG 18,551 controls	OR = 1.50 $P = 5.36 \times 10^{-9}$	[55]	Chinese 1397 PACS 943 controls	OR = 2.36 $P = 0.002$	[56]	OR = 1.59; $P = 1.3 \times 10^{-4}$	[10]
	rs1015213				Australian 232 PACG 288 controls Nepalese 106 PACG 204 controls	$P = 0.004$	[58]		
	rs1015213				Indian 180 PAC/PACG 411 controls	$P = 0.002$	[57]		

Gene	SNP	Sample	OR/P	Ref	Sample	OR/P	Ref
ABCC5	rs1401999	4276 PACG 18,801 controls	OR = 1.13 $P = 0.00046$	[59]			
	rs939336				Chinese 422 PACG 400 controls	OR = 1.46 $P = 0.013$	[60]
	rs1132776				Chinese 422 PACG 400 controls	$P = 0.007$, OR = 1.51	[60]
EPDR1	rs3816415	10,503 PACG 29,567 controls	OR = 1.24 $P = 3.49 \times 10^{-15}$	[61]	Chinese 1397 PACS 943 controls	OR = 1.49 $P < 0.001$	[56]
GLS3	rs736893	10,503 PACG 29,567 controls	OR = 1.18 $P = 1.15 \times 10^{-14}$	[61]	Chinese 1397 PACS 943 controls	Insignificant	[56]
FERMT2	rs7494379	10,503 PACG 29,567 controls	OR = 1.13 $P = 6.32 \times 10^{-11}$	[61]	Chinese 1397 PACS 943 controls	Insignificant	[56]
DRM2-FAM102A	rs3739821	10,503 PACG 29,567 controls	OR = 1.15 $P = 6.77 \times 10^{-12}$	[61]	Chinese 1397 PACS 943 controls	OR = 1.40 $P = 0.002$	[56]
CHAT	rs1258267	10,503 PACG 29,567 controls	OR = 1.22 $P = 3.73 \times 10^{-16}$	[61]	Chinese 1397 PACS 943 controls	Insignificant	[56]

Chinese cohort [56]. Two SNPs of high GWAS significance, rs11024102 of *PLEKHA7* and rs3753841 of *COL11A1*, were not replicated in a South Indian cohort [57]. The latter, *COL11A1* rs3753841, however, was replicated in a combined cohort of Australian Caucasians and Nepalese patients and controls but not in each individual cohort [62]. Three other GWAS significant SNPs, *GLS3* rs736893, *FERMT2* rs726893, and *GLS3* rs1258267 were also not associated with PACS in Chinese [56] (Table 15.2).

In a GWAS of ACD, genome-wide significant association was observed at an intronic SNP rs1401999 in the *ABCC5* gene [59]. This locus was also associated with an increased risk of PACG, suggesting a shared genetic component between PACG and its endophenotype. After testing tagging SNPs spanning the *PARL-ABCC5-HTR3D-HTR3C* region in 422 Chinese PACG patients and 400 controls all living in urban areas, we have recently revealed significant associations of PACG with 2 synonymous *ABCC5* SNPs, rs939336 (p.Cys594; OR = 1.46; 95% CI:1.08–1.97; *P* = 0.013;) and rs1132776 (p.Ala395; OR = 1.47; 95% CI: 1.10 to 1.95; *P* = 0.009) [60].

Among the GWAS associated genes, *PLEKHA7*, which encodes pleckstrin-homology-domain-containing protein 7, a junctional protein, was studied in cultured lens epithelial cells and iris tissue obtained from PACG patients, and non-pigmented ciliary epithelium (h-iNPCE) and primary trabecular meshwork cells [63]. The results revealed *PLEKHA7* to be a novel Rac1/Cdc42 GAP with a regulatory role of Rac1 and Cdc42 in the tight junction permeability of the blood-aqueous barrier. SNP rs11024102 disrupts *PLEKHA7* function, leading to deleterious effects in the blood-aqueous barrier integrity and likely aqueous humor outflow. This is thus a putative mechanism for PACG as caused by *PLEKHA7*.

15.7   Future Perspectives

Advancements in the knowledge of molecular genetics of a disease will benefit patients. Genes known to be causative of a disease can be studied

for genetic markers for pre-symptomatic diagnosis and prediction of prognosis. Responses to treatment can be related to genomics. For a disease causative gene, the mechanism and disruptive pathways leading to pathogenesis can be elucidated by investigating the gene functions, properties, and interaction networks. New therapeutic agents can be tested based on the pathology. For PACG, no causative gene has been identified. A number of susceptible genes, with gene variants associated with the disease, are known. But the information is yet insufficient to establish a genetic marker or to throw light to the disease mechanism. GWAS on large samples of well-characterized patients is needed to find more PACG genes. Exome sequencing and whole-genome sequencing together with family linkage and sibling pair studies should help to identify more PACG genes and sequence variants that are responsible for the disease development.

Acknowledgments This work was supported in part by research grants 14100917 (C.P.P.) from the General Research Fund, Hong Kong; research grants 01122236, 11120801 and 07180256 (L.J.C.) from the Health and Medical Research Fund, Hong Kong; and the Endowment Fund for Lim Por-Yen Eye Genetics Research Centre, Hong Kong.

Compliance with Ethical RequirementsLi Jia Chen, Shi Song Rong, and Chi Pui Pang declare that they have no conflict of interest. No human or animal studies were performed by the authors for this article.

References

1. Quigley HA. Angle-closure Glaucoma – simpler answers to complex mechanisms. Am J Ophthalmol. 2009;148:657–69.
2. Sundin OH, Leppert GS, Silva ED, Yang JM, Dharmaraj S, Maumenee IH, Santos LC, Parsa CF, Traboulsi EI, Broman KW, Dibernardo C, Sunness JS, Toy J, Weinberg EM. Extreme hyperopia is the result of null mutations in MFRP, which encodes a frizzled-related protein. Proc Natl Acad Sci U S A. 2005;102:9553–8.
3. Nongpiur ME, Ku JY, Aung T. Angle closure glaucoma: a mechanistic review. Curr Opin Ophthalmol. 2011;22:96–101.
4. Ritch R. Plateau iris is caused by abnormally positioned ciliary processes. J Glaucoma. 1992;1:23–6.

5. Carricondo PC, Andrade T, Prasov L, Ayres BM, Moroi SE. Nanophthalmos: a review of the clinical Spectrum and genetics. J Ophthalmol. 2018;2018:2735465.

6. Salmon JF. Predisposing factors for chronic angle-closure glaucoma. Prog Retinal Eye Res. 1998;18:121.

7. Wang X, Liu X, Huang L, Fang S, Jia X, Xiao X, Li S, Guo X. Mutation survey of candidate genes and genotype-phenotype analysis in 20 southeastern Chinese patients with Axenfeld-Rieger syndrome. Curr Eye Res. 2018 Nov;43(11):1334–41.

8. Wiggs JL, Pasquale LR. Genetics of glaucoma. Hum Mol Genet. 2017;26:R21–7.

9. Ahram DF, Alward WL, Kuehn MH. The genetic mechanisms of primary angle closure glaucoma. Eye (Lond). 2015;29:1251–9.

10. Rong SS, Tang FY, Chu WK, Ma L, Yam JC, Tang SM, Li J, Gu H, Young AL, Tham CC, Pang CP, Chen LJ. Genetic associations of primary angle-closure disease: a systematic review and Meta-analysis. Ophthalmology. 2016;123:1211–21.

11. Aung T, Khor CC. Glaucoma genetics: recent advances and future directions. Asia Pacific J Ophthalmol. 2016;5:256–9.

12. Alsbirk PH. Primary angle-closure glaucoma. Oculometry, epidemiology, and genetics in a high risk population. Acta Ophthalmol Suppl. 1976;127:5–31.

13. Alsbirk PH. Variation and heritability of ocular dimensions. A population study among adult Greenland Eskimos. Acta Ophthalmol. 1977;55:443–56.

14. Day AC, Baio G, Gazzard G, Bunce C, Azuara-Blanco A, Munoz B, Friedman DS, Foster PJ. The prevalence of primary angle closure glaucoma in European derived populations: a systematic review. Br J Ophthalmol. 2012;96:1162–7.

15. Tham YC, Li X, Wong TY, Quigley HA, Aung T, Cheng CY. Global prevalence of glaucoma and projections of glaucoma burden through 2040: a systematic review and meta-analysis. Ophthalmology. 2014;121:2081–90.

16. Chan EW, Li X, Tham YC, Liao J, Wong TY, Aung T, Cheng CY. Glaucoma in Asia: regional prevalence variations and future projections. Br J Ophthalmol. 2016;100:78–85.

17. Paul C, Sengupta S, Banerjee S, Choudbury S. Angle closure glaucoma in rural and urban populations in eastern India – the Hooghly River Glaucoma study. Indian J Ophthalmol. 2018;66:1285–90.

18. Cheng JW, Cheng SW, Ma XY, Cai JP, Li Y, Wei RL. The prevalence of primaryglaucoma in mainland China: a systematic review and meta-analysis. J Glaucoma. 2013;22:301–6.

19. Song P, Wang J, Bucan K, Theodoratou E, Rudan I, Chan KY. National and subnational prevalence and burden of glaucoma in China: a systematic analysis. J Glob Health. 2017;7:020705.

20. Liang Y, Friedman DS, Zhou Q, Yang XH, Sun LP, Guo L, Chang DS, Lian L, Wang NL. Handan eye study group. Prevalance and characteristics of primary angle-closure diseases in a rural adult Chinese population: the Handan eye study. Invest Ophthalmol Vis Sci. 2011;52:8672–9.

21. He M, Foster PJ, Ge J, Huang W, Zheng Y, Friedman DS, Lee PS, Khaw PT. Prevalence and clinical characteristics of glaucoma in adult Chinese: a population-based study in Liwan District. Guangzhou Invest Ophthalmol Vis Sci. 2006;47:2782–8.

22. Lowe RF. Primary angle closure glaucoma. Family histories and anterior chamber depths. Br J Ophthalmol. 1964;48:191–5.

23. Leighton DA. Survey of the first-degree relatives of glaucoma patients. Trans Ophthalmol Soc U K. 1976;96:28–32.

24. Amerasinghe N, Zhang J, Thalamuthu A, He M, Vithana EN, Viswanathan A, Wong TY, Foster PJ, Aung T. The heritability and sibling risk of angle closure in Asians. Ophthalmology. 2011;118:480–5.

25. Kavitha S, Zebardast N, Palaniswamy K, Wojciechowski R, Chan ES, Friedman DS, Venkatesh R, Ramulu PY. Family history is a strong risk factor for prevalent angle closure in a south Indian population. Ophthalmology. 2014;121:2091–7.

26. Zebardast N, Kavitha S, Palaniswamy K, Sengupta S, Kader MA, Raman G, Reddy S, Ramulu PY, Venkatesh R. Angle closure phenotypes in siblings of patients at different stages of angle closure. Ophthalmology. 2016;123:1622–4.

27. Yazdani S, Akbarian S, Pakravan M, Afrouzifar M. Prevalence of angle closure in siblings of patients with primary angle-closure glaucoma. J Glaucoma. 2015;24:149–53.

28. Klein BE, Klein R, Lee KE. Heritability of risk factors for primary open-angle glaucoma: the beaver dam eye study. Invest Ophthalmol Vis Sci. 2004;45:59–62.

29. Chang TC, Congdon NG, Wojciechowski R, Muñoz B, Gilbert D, Chen P, Friedman DS, West SK. Determinants and heritability of intraocular pressure and cup-to-disc ratio in a defined older population. Ophthalmology. 2005;112:1186–91.

30. He M, Liu B, Huang W, Zhang J, Yin Q, Zheng Y, Wang D, Ge J. Heritability of optic disc and cup measured by the Heidelberg retinal tomography in Chinese: the Guangzhou twin eye study. Invest Ophthalmol Vis Sci. 2008;49:1350–5.

31. He M, Ge J, Wang D, Zhang J, Hewitt AW, Hur YM, Mackey DA, Foster PJ. Heritability of the iridotrabecular angle width measured by optical ccherence tomography in Chinese children: the Guangzhou twin eye study. Invest Ophthalmol Vis Sci. 2008;49:1356–61.

32. Tu YS, Yin ZQ, Pen HM, Yuan CM. Genetic heritability of a shallow anterior chamber in Chinese families with primary angle closure glaucoma. Ophthalmic Genet. 2008;29:171–6.

33. Zhuang W, Wang S, Hao J, Xu M, Chi H, Piao S, Ma J, Zhang X, Ha S. Genotype-ocular biometry correlation analysis of eight primary angle closure glaucoma susceptibility loci in a cohort from northern China. PLoS One. 2018;13:e0206935.

34. Wang S, Zhuang W, Ma J, Xu M, Piao S, Hao J, Zhang W, Chi H, Xue Z, Ha S. Association of Genes

implicated in primary angle-closure Glaucoma and the ocular biometric parameters of anterior chamber depth and axial length in a northern Chinese population. BMC Ophthalmol. 2018;18:271.

35. Day AC, Luben R, Khawaja AP, Low S, Hayat S, Dalzell N, Wareham NJ, Khaw KT, Foster PJ. Genotype-phenotype analysis of SNPs associated with primary angle closure glaucoma (rs1015213, rs3753841 and rs11024102) and ocular biometry in the EPIC-Norfolk eye study. Br J Ophthalmol. 2013;97:704–7.

36. Khawaja AP, Chan MPY, Yip JLY, Broadway DC, Garway-Heath DF, Viswanathan AC, Luben R, Hayat S, Hauser MA, Wareham NJ, Khaw KT, Fortune B, Allingham RR, Foster PJ. A common Glaucoma-risk variant of SIX6 alters retinal nerve Fiber layer and optic disc measures in a European population: the EPIC-Norfolk eye study. J Glaucoma. 2018;27: 743–9.

37. Cheng CY, Allingham RR, Aung T, Tham YC, Hauser MA, Vithana EN, Khor CC, Wong TY. Association of common SIX6 polymorphisms with peripapillary retinal nerve fiber layer thickness: the Singapore Chinese eye study. Invest Ophthalmol Vis Sci. 2014;56:478–83.

38. Gasten AC, Ramdas WD, Broer L, van Koolwijk LM, Ikram MK, de Jong PT, Aulchenko YS, Wolfs RC, Hofman A, Rivadeneira F, Uitterlinden AG, Oostra BA, Lemij HG, Klaver CC, Jansonius NM, Vingerling JR, van Duijn CM. A genetic epidemiologic study of candidate genes involved in the optic nerve head morphology. Invest Ophthalmol Vis Sci. 2012;53:1485–91.

39. Ramdas WD, van Koolwijk LM, Ikram MK, Jansonius NM, de Jong PT, Bergen AA, Isaacs A, Amin N, Aulchenko YS, Wolfs RC, Hofman A, Rivadeneira F, Oostra BA, Uitterlinden AG, Hysi P, Hammond CJ, Lemij HG, Vingerling JR, Klaver CC, van Duijn CM. A genome-wide association study of optic disc parameters. PLoS Genet. 2010;6:e1000978.

40. Micheal S, Qamar R, Akhtar F, Khan MI, Khan WA, Ahmed A. MTHFR gene C677T and A1298C polymorphisms and homocysteine levels in primary open angle and primaryclosed angle glaucoma. Mol Vis. 2009;15:2268–78.

41. Shi H, Zhang J, Zhu R, Hu N, Lu H, Yang M, Qin B, Shi J, Guan H. Primary angle closure and sequence variants within MicroRNA binding sites of genes involved in eye development. PLoS One. 2016;11:e0166055.

42. Chakrabarti S, Devi KR, Komatireddy S, Kaur K, Parikh RS, Mandal AK, Chandrasekhar G, Thomas R. Glaucoma-associated CYP1B1 mutations share similar haplotype backgrounds in POAG and PACG phenotypes. Invest Ophthalmol Vis Sci. 2007;48:5439–44.

43. Awadalla MS, Burdon KP, Thapa SS, Hewitt AW, Craig JE. A cross-ethnicity investigation of genes previously implicated in primary angle closure glaucoma. Mol Vis. 2012;18:2247–54.

44. Cao D, Liu X, Guo X, Cong Y, Huang J, Mao Z. Investigation of the association between CALCRL polymorphisms and primary angle closure glaucoma. Mol Vis. 2009;15:2202–8.

45. Awadalla MS, Thapa SS, Burdon KP, Hewitt AW, Craig JE. The association of hepatocyte growth factor (HGF) gene with primary angle closure glaucoma in the Nepalese population. Mol Vis. 2011;17:2248–54.

46. Ayub H, Khan MI, Micheal S, Akhtar F, Ajmal M, Shafique S, Ali SH, den Hollander AI, Ahmed A, Qamar R. Association of eNOS and HSP70 gene polymorphisms with glaucoma in Pakistani cohorts. Mol Vis. 2010;16:18–25.

47. Awadalla MS, Thapa SS, Hewitt AW, Craig JE, Burdon KP. Association of eNOSpolymorphisms with primary angle-closure glaucoma. Invest Ophthalmol Vis Sci. 2013;54:2108–14.

48. Shi H, Zhu R, Hu N, Shi J, Zhang J, Jiang L, Jiang H, Guan H. Association of frizzled-related protein (MFRP) and heat shock protein 70 (HSP70) single-nucleotide polymorphisms with primary angle closure in a Han Chinese population: Jiangsu eye study. Mol Vis. 2013;19:128–34.

49. Awadalla MS, Burdon KP, Kuot A, Hewitt AW, Craig JE. Matrix metalloproteinase-9 genetic variation and primary angle closure glaucoma in a Caucasian population. Mol Vis. 2011;17:1420–4.

50. Wang IJ, Chiang TH, Shih YF, Lu SC, Lin LL, Shieh JW, Wang TH, Samples JR, Hung PT. The association of single nucleotide polymorphisms in the MMP-9 genes with susceptibility to acute primary angle closure glaucoma in Taiwanese patients. Mol Vis. 2006;12:1223–32.

51. Cong Y, Guo X, Liu X, Cao D, Jia X, Xiao X, Li S, Fang S, Zhang Q. Association of the single nucleotide polymorphisms in the extracellular matrix metalloprotease-9 gene with PACG in southern China. Mol Vis. 2009;15:1412–7.

52. Micheal S, Yousaf S, Khan MI, Akhtar F, Islam F, Khan WA, den Hollander AI, Qamar R. Ahmed a polymorphisms in matrix metalloproteinases MMP1 and MMP9 are associated with primary open-angle and angle closure glaucoma in a Pakistani population. Mol Vis. 2013;19:441–7.

53. Suri F, Yazdani S, Chapi M, Safari I, Rasooli P, Daftarian N, Jafarinasab MR, Ghasemi Firouzabadi S, Alehabib E, Darvish H, Klotzle B, Fan JB, Turk C. Elahi E.COL18A1 is a candidate eye iridocorneal angle-closure gene in humans. Hum Mol Genet. 2018;27:3772–86.

54. Jeoung JW, Ko JH, Kim YJ, Kim YW, Park KH, Oh JY. Microarray-based analysis of gene expression profiles in peripheral blood of patients with acute primary angle closure. Ophthalmic Genet. 2017;38:520–6.

55. Vithana EN, Khor CC, Qiao C, Nongpiur ME, George R, Chen LJ, Do T, Abu-Amero K, Huang CK, Low S, Tajudin LA, Perera SA, Cheng CY, Xu L, Jia H, Ho CL, Sim KS, Wu RY, CCY T, PTK C, Su DH, Oen FT, Sarangapani S, Soumittra N, Osman EA, Wong HT, Tang G, Fan S, Meng H, DTL H, Wang

H, Feng B, Baskaran M, Shantha B, Ramprasad VL, Kumaramanickavel G, Iyengar SK, How AC, Lee KY, Sivakumaran TA, VHK Y, SML T, Li Y, Wang YX, Tay WT, Sim X, Lavanya R, Cornes BK, Zheng YF, Wong TT, Loon SC, VKY Y, Waseem N, Yaakub A, Chia KS, Allingham RR, Hauser MA, DSC L, Hibberd ML, Bhattacharya SS, Zhang M, Teo YY, Tan DT, Jonas JB, Tai ES, Saw SM, Hon DN, Al-Obeidan SA, Liu J, TNB C, Simmons CP, Bei JX, Zeng YX, Foster PJ, Vijaya L, Wong TY, Pang CP, Wang N, Aung T. Genome-wide association analyses identify three new susceptibility loci for primary angle closure glaucoma. Nat Genet. 2012;44:1142–6.

56. Nongpiur ME, Cheng CY, Duvesh R, Vijayan S, Baskaran M, Khor CC, Allen J, Kavitha S, Venkatesh R, Goh D, Husain R, Boey PY, Quek D, Ho CL, Wong TT, Perera S, Wong TY, Krishnadas SR, Sundaresan P, Aung T, Vithana EN. Evaluation of primary angle-closure Glaucoma susceptibility loci in patients with early stages of angle-closure disease. Ophthalmology. 2018;125:664–70.

57. Duvesh R, Verma A, Venkatesh R, Kavitha S, Ramulu PY, Wojciechowski R, Sundaresan P. Association study in a south Indian population supports rs1015213 as a risk factor for primary angle closure. Invest Ophthalmol Vis Sci. 2013;54:5624–8.

58. Awadalla MS, Thapa SS, Hewitt AW, Burdon KP, Craig JE. Association of genetic variants with primary angle closure glaucoma in two different populations. PLoS One. 2013;8:e67903.

59. Nongpiur ME, Khor CC, Jia H, Cornes BK, Chen LJ, Qiao C, Nair KS, Cheng CY, Xu L, George R, Tan D, Abu-Amero K, Perera SA, Ozaki M, Mizoguchi T, Kurimoto Y, Low S, Tajudin LS, Ho CL, Tham CC, Soto I, Chew PT, Wong HT, Shantha B, Kuroda M, Osman EA, Tang G, Fan S, Meng H, Wang H, Feng B, Yong VH, Ting SM, Li Y, Wang YX, Li Z, Lavanya R, Wu RY, Zheng YF, Su DH, Loon SC, Yong VK, Allingham RR, Hauser MA, Soumittra N, Ramprasad VL, Waseem N, Yaakub A, Chia KS, Kumaramanickavel G, Wong TT, How AC, Chau TN, Simmons CP, Bei JX, Zeng YX, Bhattacharya SS, Zhang M, Tan DT, Teo YY, Al-Obeidan SA, Hon DN, Tai ES, Saw SM, Foster PJ, Vijaya L, Jonas JB, Wong TY, John SW, Pang CP, Vithana EN, Wang N, Aung T. ABCC5, a gene that influences the anterior chamber depth, is associated with primary angle closure glaucoma. PLoS Genet. 2014;10:e1004089.

60. Tang FY, Ma L, Tam POS, Pang CP, Tham CC, Chen LJ. Genetic association of the PARL-ABCC5-HTR3D-HTR3C locus with primary angle-closure Glaucoma in Chinese. Invest Ophthalmol Vis Sci. 2017;58:4384–9.

61. Khor CC, Do T, Jia H, Nakano M, George R, Abu-Amero K, Duvesh R, Chen LJ, Li Z, Nongpiur ME, Perera SA, Qiao C, Wong HT, Sakai H, Barbosa de Melo M, Lee MC, Chan AS, Azhany Y, Dao TL, Ikeda Y, Perez-Grossmann RA, Zarnowski T, Day AC, Jonas JB, Tam PO, Tran TA, Ayub H, Akhtar F, Micheal S,

Chew PT, Aljasim LA, Dada T, Luu TT, Awadalla MS, Kitnarong N, Wanichwecharungruang B, Aung YY, Mohamed-Noor J, Vijayan S, Sarangapani S, Husain R, Jap A, Baskaran M, Goh D, Su DH, Wang H, Yong VK, Yip LW, Trinh TB, Makornwattana M, Nguyen TT, Leuenberger EU, Park KH, Wiyogo WA, Kumar RS, Tello C, Kurimoto Y, Thapa SS, Pathanapitoon K, Salmon JF, Sohn YH, Fea A, Ozaki M, Lai JS, Tantisevi V, Khaing CC, Mizoguchi T, Nakano S, Kim CY, Tang G, Fan S. Wu R, Meng H, Nguyen TT, Tran TD, Ueno M, Martinez JM, Ramli N, Aung YM, Reyes RD, Vernon SA, Fang SK, Xie Z, Chen XY, Foo JN, Sim KS, Wong TT, Quek DT, Venkatesh R, Kavitha S, Krishnadas SR, Soumittra N, Shantha B, Lim BA, Ogle J, de Vasconcellos JP, Costa VP, Abe RY, de Souza BB, Sng CC, Aquino MC, Kosior-Jarecka E, Fong GB, Tamanaja VC, Fujita R, Jiang Y, Waseem N, Low S, Pham HN, Al-Shahwan S, Craven ER, Khan MI, Dada R, Mohanty K, Faiq MA, Hewitt AW, Burdon KP, Gan EH, Prutthipongsit A, Patthanathamrongkasem T, Catacutan MA, Felarca IR, Liao CS, Rusmayani E, Istiantoro VW, Consolandi G, Pignata G, Lavia C, Rojanapongpun P, Mangkornkanokpong L, Chansangpetch S, Chan JC, Choy BN, Shum JW, Than HM, Oo KT, Han AT, Yong VH, Ng XY, Goh SR, Chong YF, Hibberd ML, Seielstad M, Png E, Dunstan SJ, Chau NV, Bei J, Zeng YX, Karkey A, Basnyat B, Pasutto F, Paoli D, Frezzotti P, Wang JJ, Mitchell P, Fingert JH, Allingham RR, Hauser MA, Lim ST, Chew SH, Ebstein RP, Sakuntabhai A, Park KH, Ahn J, Boland G, Snippe H, Stead R, Quino R, Zaw SN, Lukasik U, Shetty R, Zahari M, Bae HW, Oo NL, Kubota T, Manassakorn A, Ho WL, Dallorto L, Hwang YH, Kiire CA, Kuroda M, Djamal ZE, Peregrino JI, Ghosh A, Jeoung JW, Hoan TS, Srisamran N, Sandragasu T, Set SH, Doan VH, Bhattacharya SS, Ho CL, Tan DT, Sihota R, Loon SC, Mori K, Kinoshita S, Hollander AI, Qamar R, Wang YX, Teo YY, Tai ES, Hartleben-Matkin C, Lozano-Giral D, Saw SM, Cheng CY, Zenteno JC, Pang CP, Bui HT, Hee O, Craig JE, Edward DP, Yonahara M, Neto JM, Guevara-Fujita ML, Xu L, Ritch R, Liza-Sharmin AT, Wong TY, Al-Obeidan S, Do NH SP, Tham CC, Foster PJ, Vijaya L, Tashiro K, Vithana EN, Wang N, Aung T. Genome-wide association study identifies five new susceptibility loci for primary angle closure glaucoma. Nat Genet. 2016;48:556–62.

62. Awadalla MS, Thapa SS, Hewitt AW, Burdon KP, Craig JE. Association of genetic variants with primary angle closure glaucoma in two different populations. PLoS One. 2013;8:e67903.

63. Lee MC, Shei W, Chan AS, Chua BT, Goh SR, Chong YF, Hilmy MH, Nongpiur ME, Baskaran M, Khor CC, Aung T, Hunziker W, Vithana EN. Primary angle closure glaucoma (PACG) susceptibility gene PLEKHA7 encodes a novel Rac1/Cdc42 GAP that modulates cell migration and blood-aqueous barrier function. Hum Mol Genet. 2017;26:4011–27.